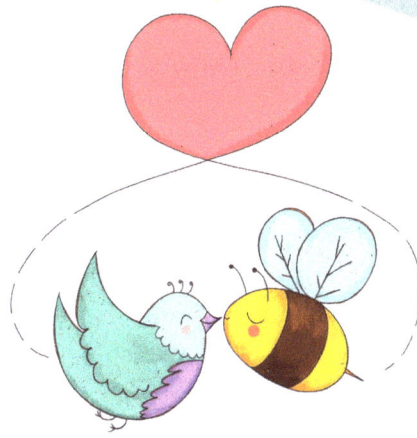

## PAPERDOLL PLAY & LEARN

# WHERE DO BABIES COME FROM?

## LEARN ABOUT PREGNANCY, BIRTH AND BABIES

By Cath Hakanson

Illustrated by Embla Granqvist

# PAPERDOLL PLAY & LEARN
# WHERE DO BABIES COME FROM?

by Cath Hakanson

Published by Sex Ed Rescue

PO Box 7903 | Cloisters Square WA 6850 | Australia

sexedrescue.com

Illustrated by Embla Granqvist

Clothing illustrated by Moch. Fajar Shobaru

Cover and interior design by Jevgenija Bitter

For permission contact:
cath@sexedrescue.com

ISBN-13: 978-0-6487162-3-5

# INSTRUCTIONS

**1.** Color in the dolls and clothes before cutting out.

**2.** For best results, glue the doll and stand to cardboard with a gluestick and allow to dry before cutting.

**3.** Carefully cut out dolls and stand with sharp scissors.

**4.** Cut along dotted line on both the stand and the doll base.

**5.** Insert the stand onto the base.

**6.** Cut out the clothes. Fold tabs over, slip tabs behind doll to fit. Clothes will fit all dolls.

**TIP** An alternative method to attach clothes (with no tabs) is to use Scotch® Restickable Strips. Attach half a sticky strip to the doll and clothes will be easy to change, with no more torn tabs and clothes

For more hours of imaginative play and fun, you can download some coloring in about babies for your child to play with at HTTPS://SEXEDRESCUE.COM/BABIES/

# ROWAN

## NEWBORN

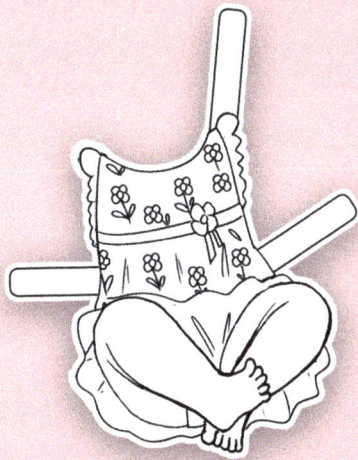

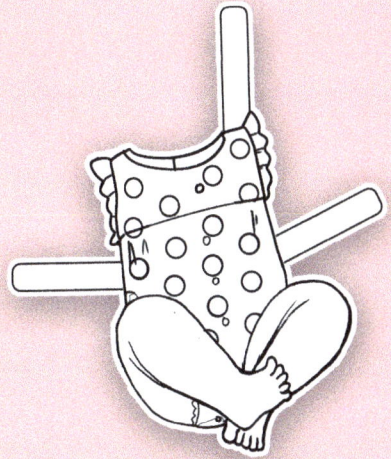

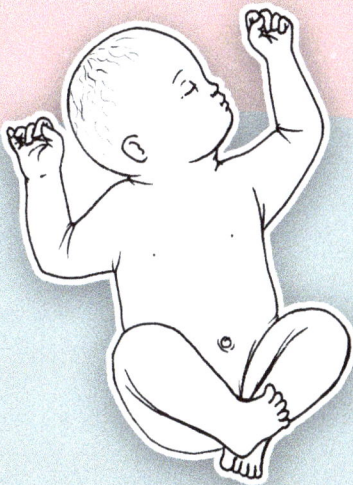

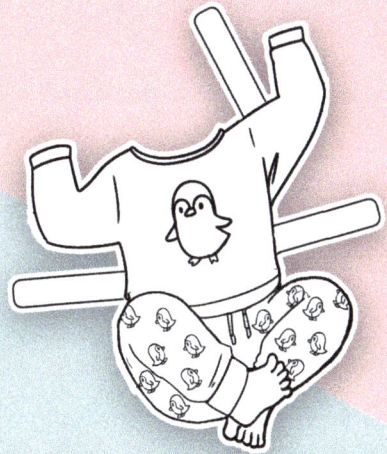

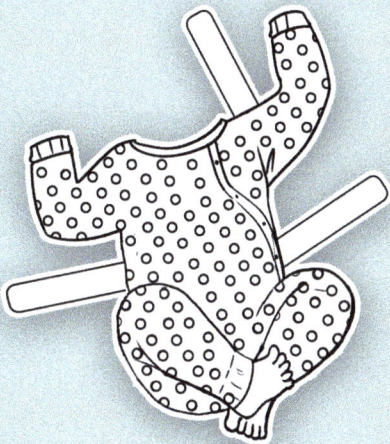

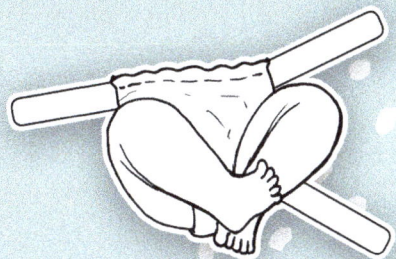

# BILLIE

## 3 MONTHS OLD

ROWAN

ROWAN

ROWAN

ROWAN

ROWAN

ROWAN

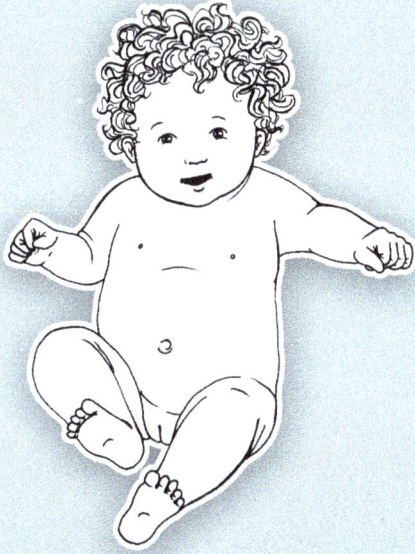

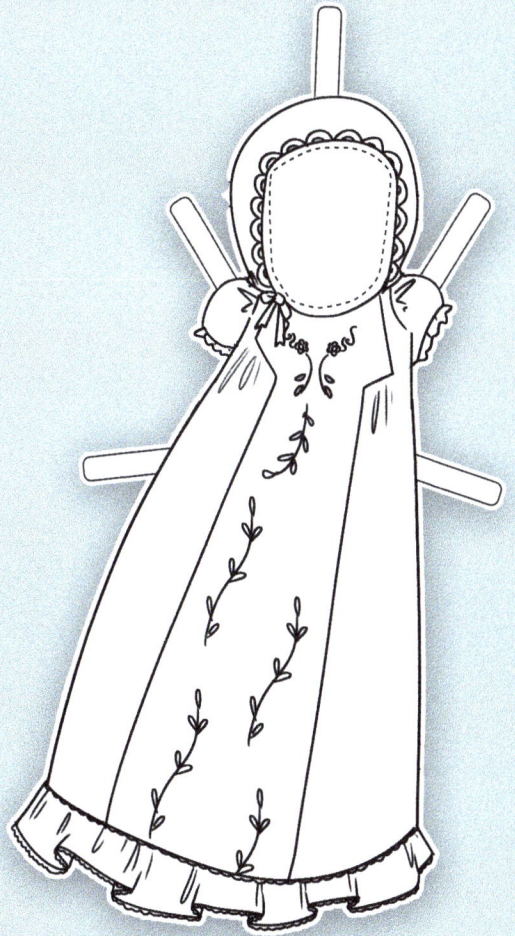

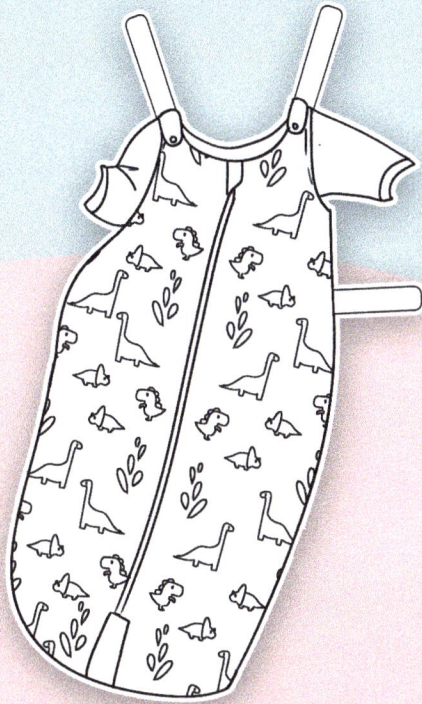

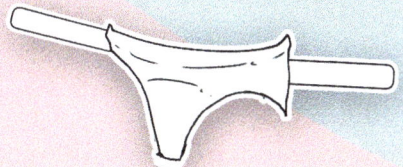

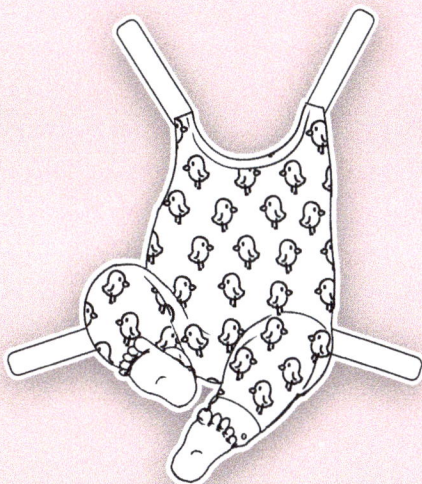

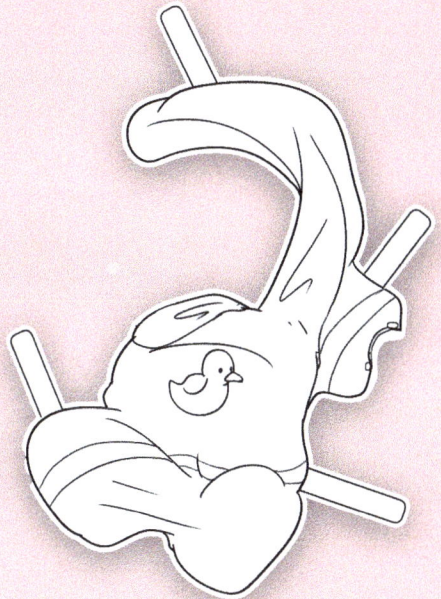

# JESSIE

## 6 MONTHS OLD

BILLIE

BILLIE

BILLIE

BILLIE

BILLIE

BILLIE

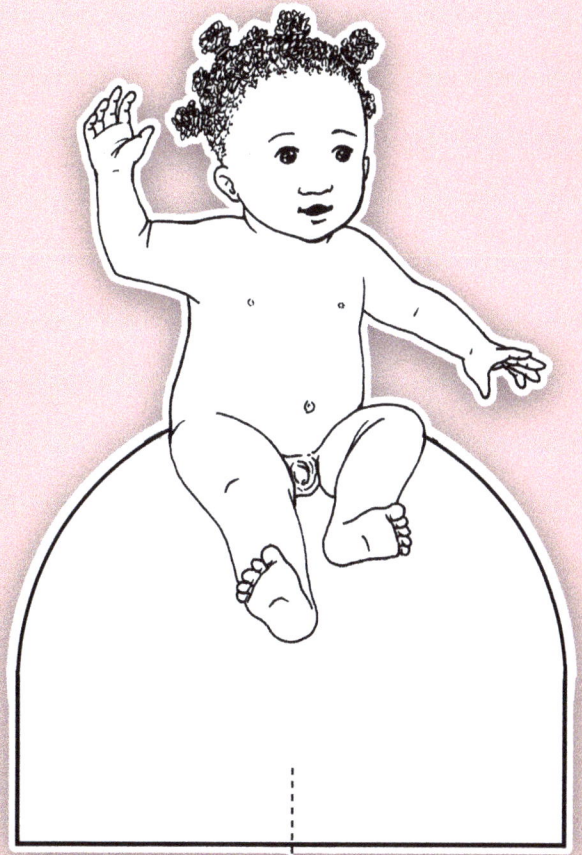

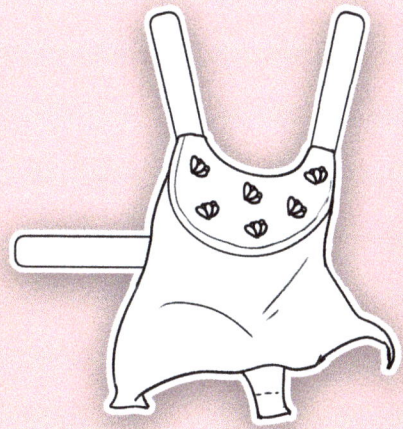

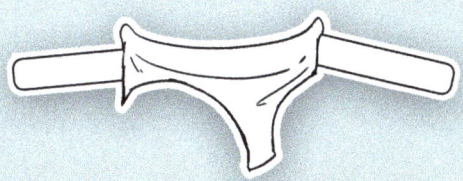

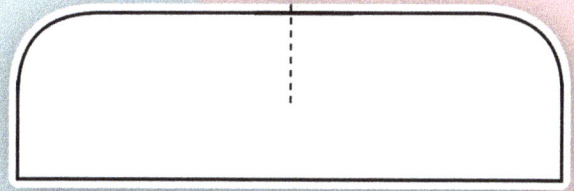

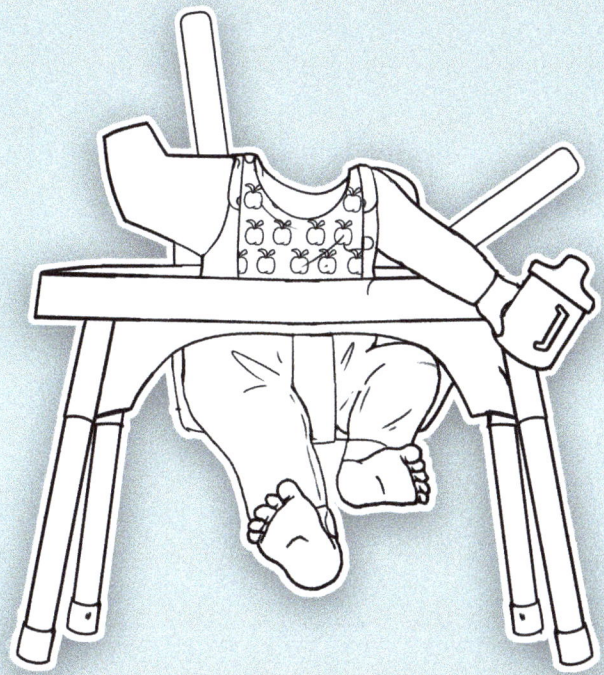

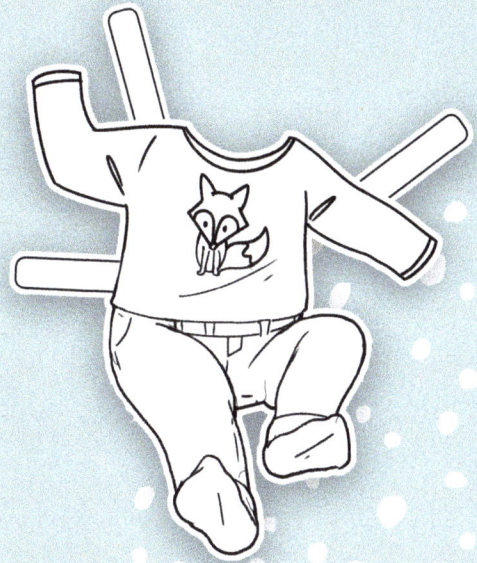

# GEORGIE

## 9 MONTHS OLD

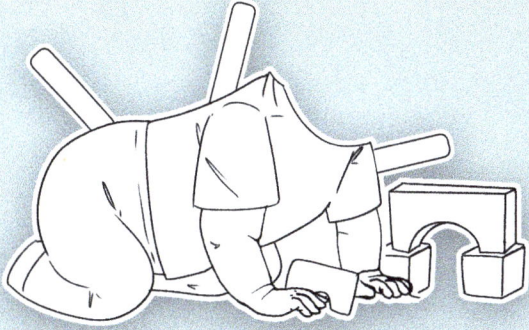

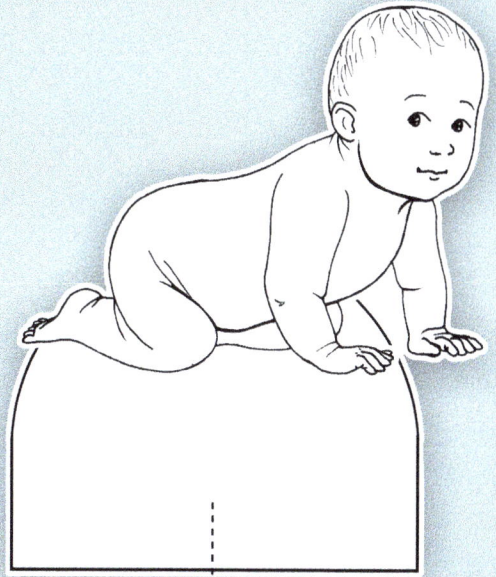

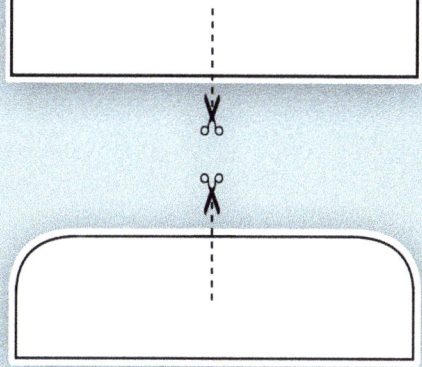

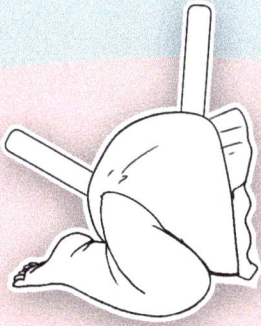

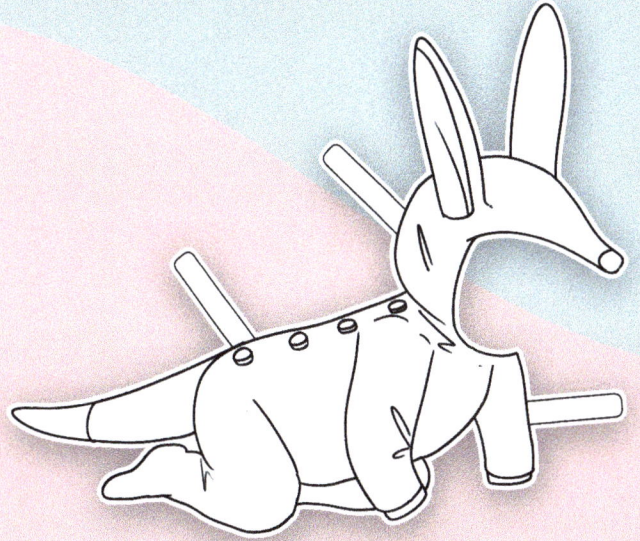

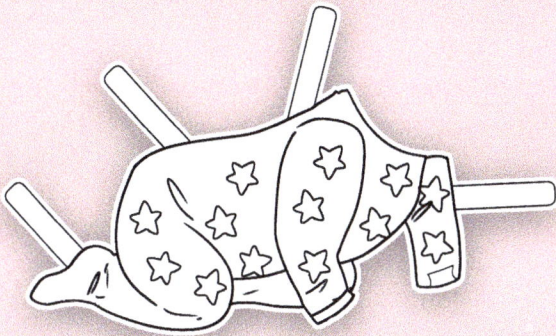

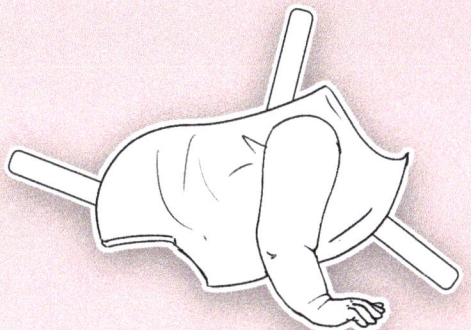

# CHARLIE

## 12 MONTHS OLD

GEORGIE

GEORGIE

GEORGIE

GEORGIE

GEORGIE

GEORGIE

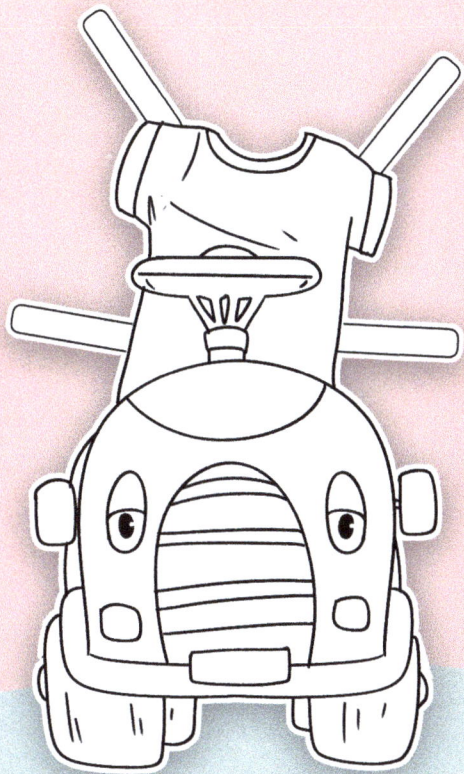

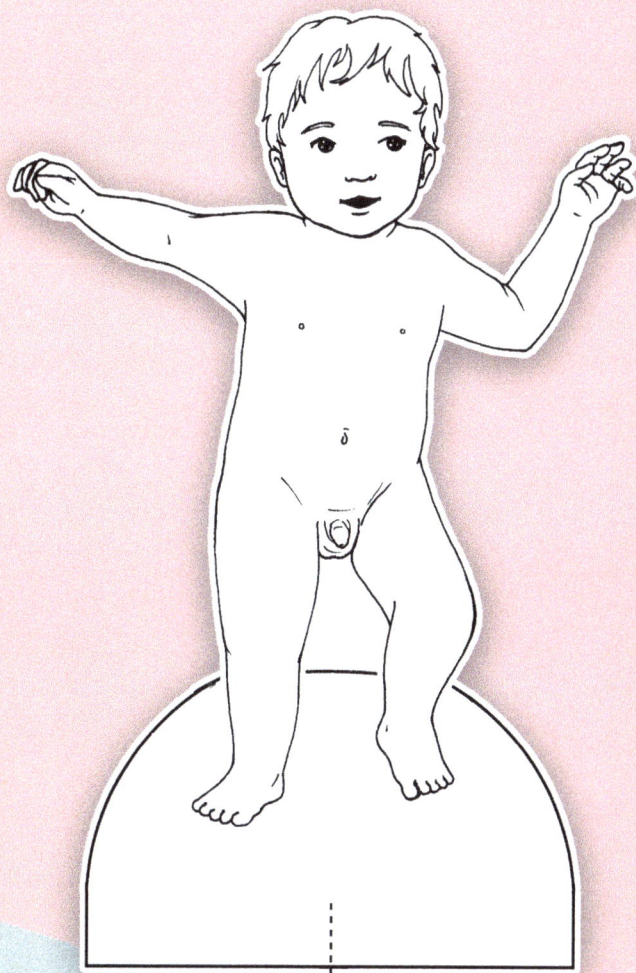

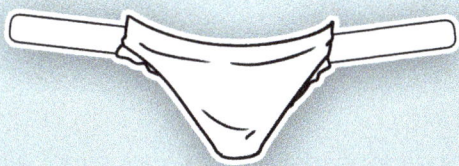

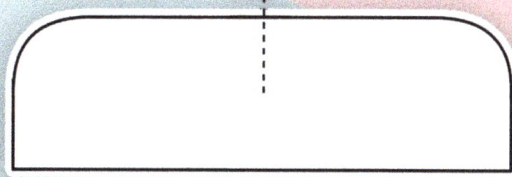

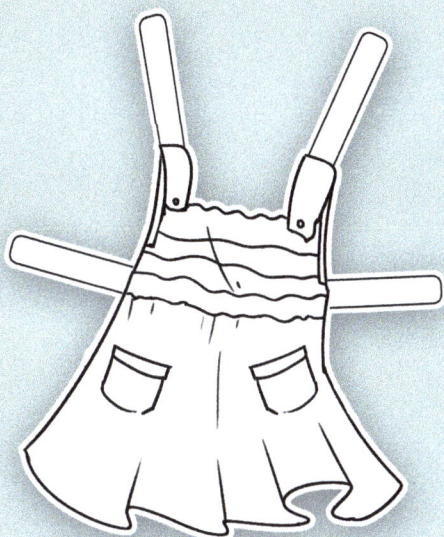

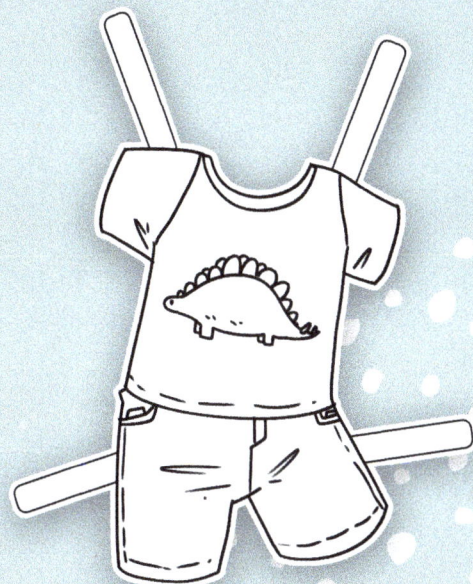

# SAM

## 18 MONTHS OLD

CHARLIE

CHARLIE

CHARLIE

CHARLIE

CHARLIE

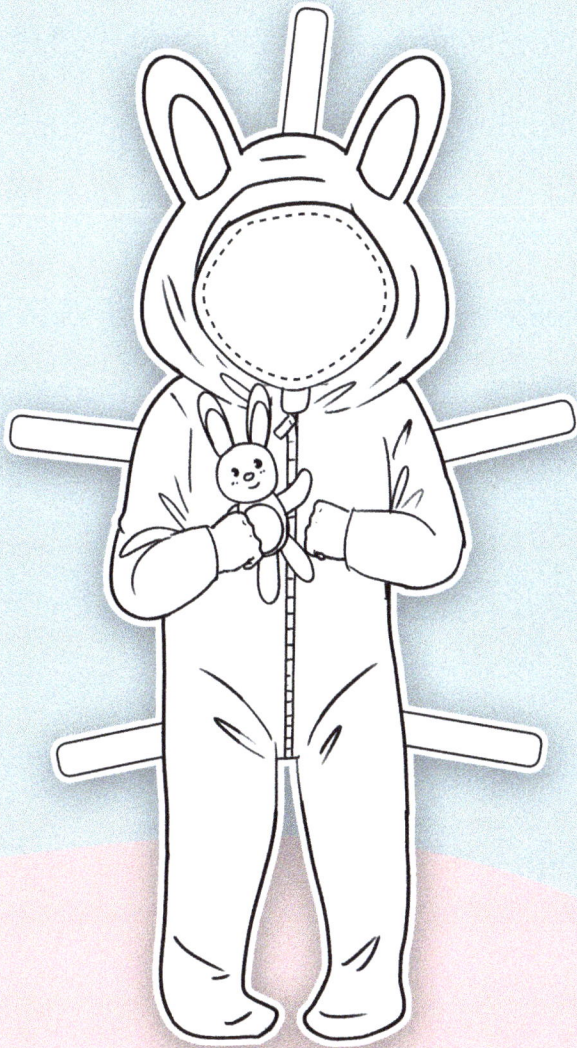

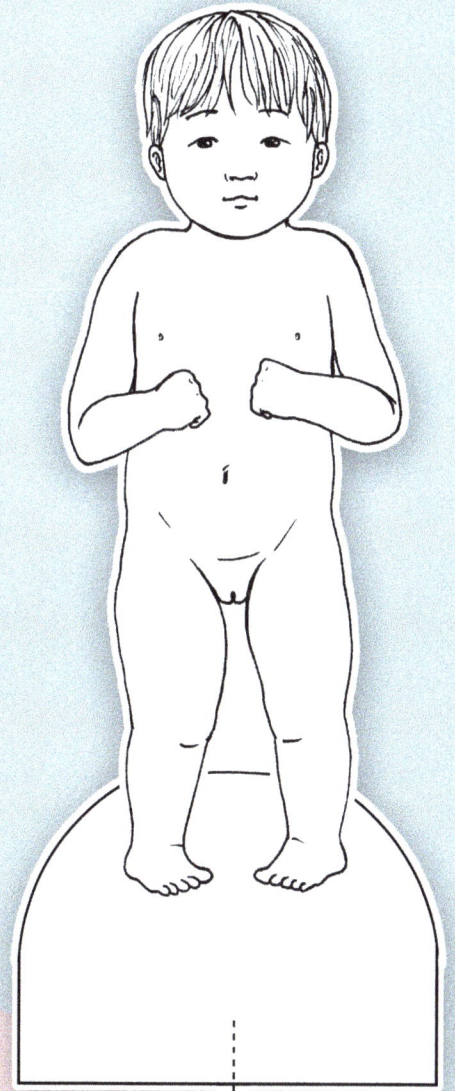

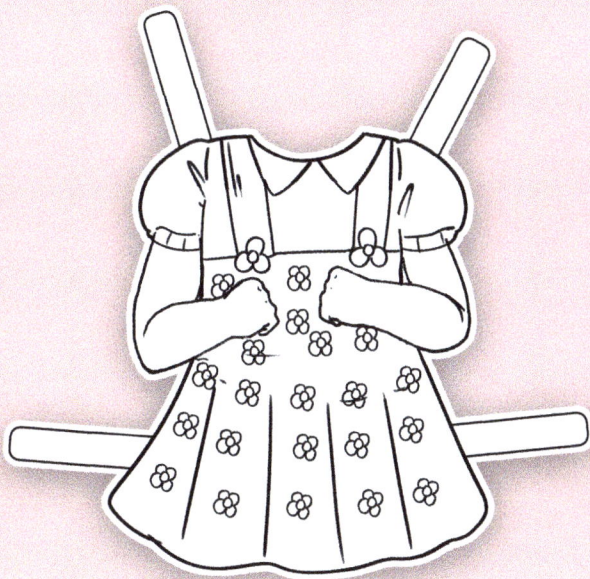

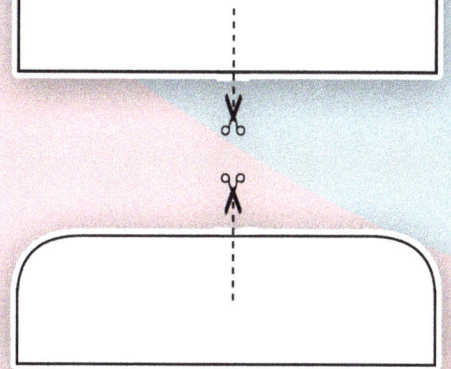

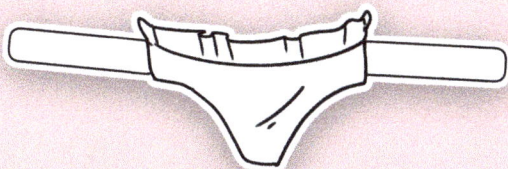

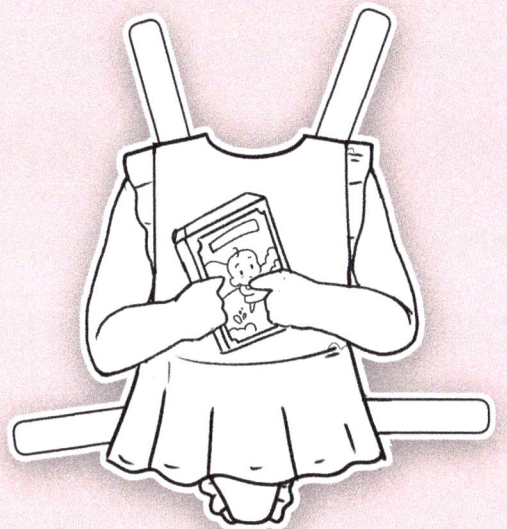

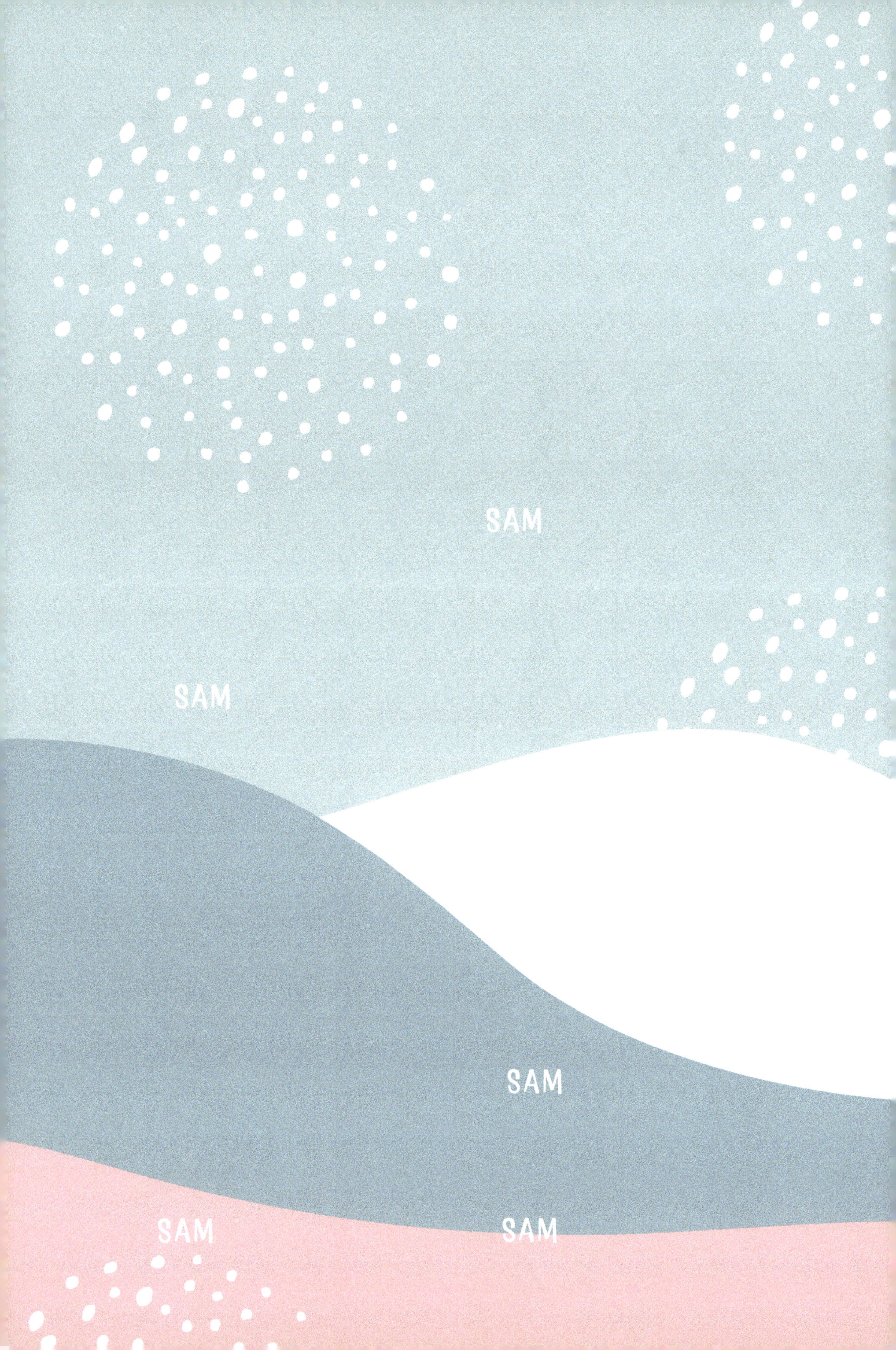

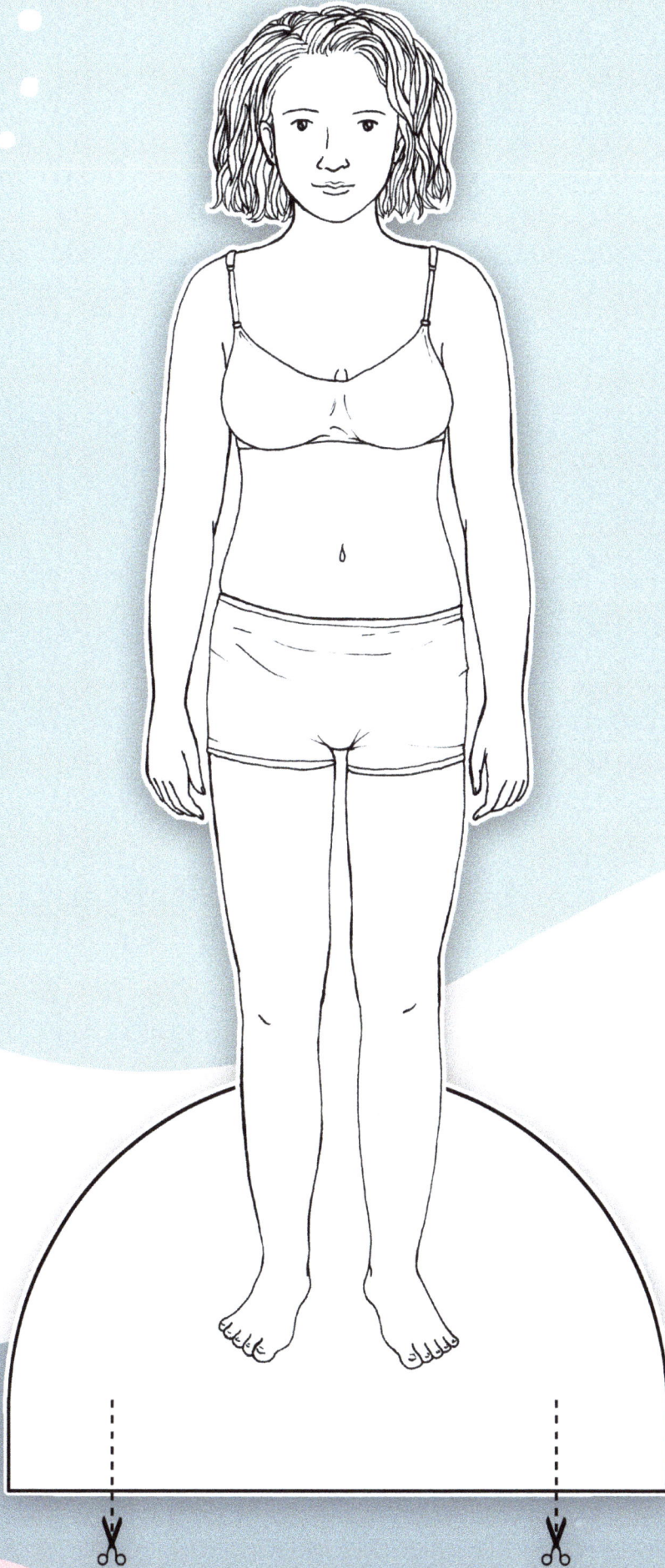

JO

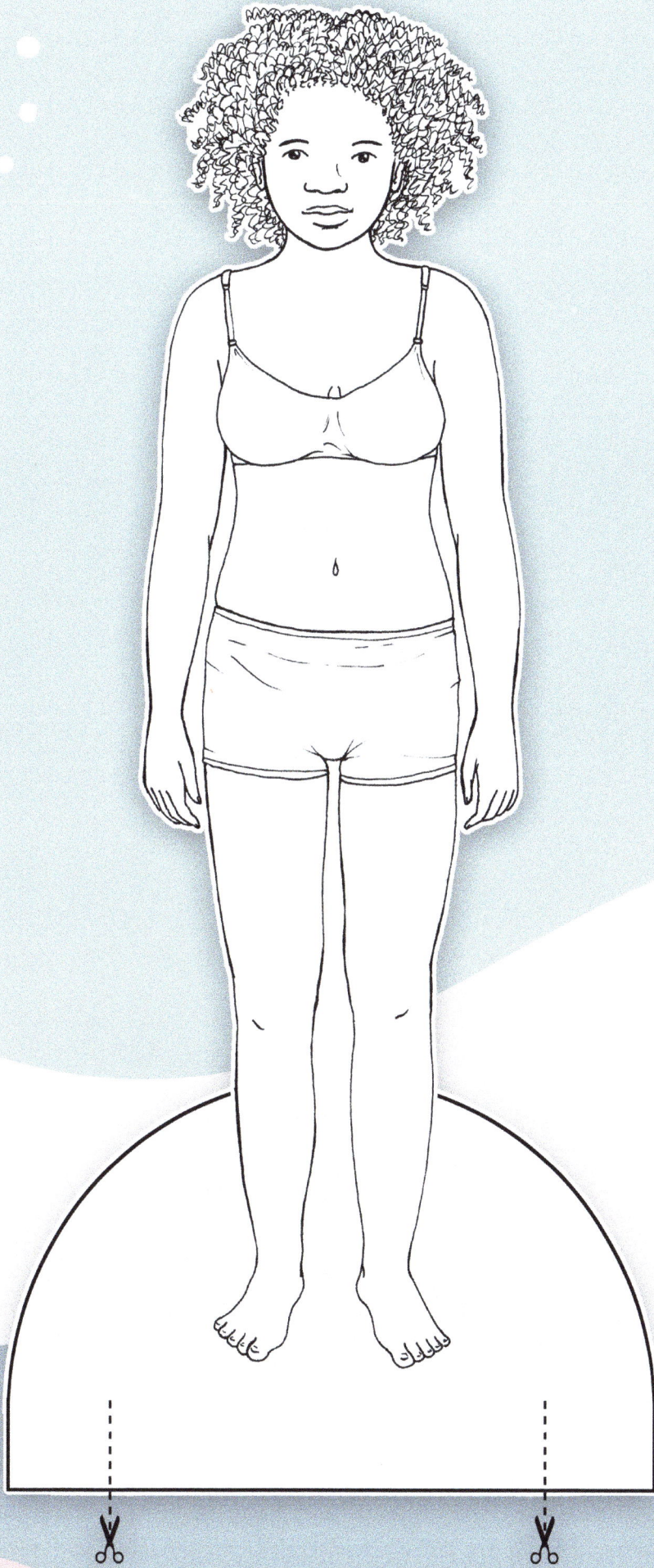

LOU

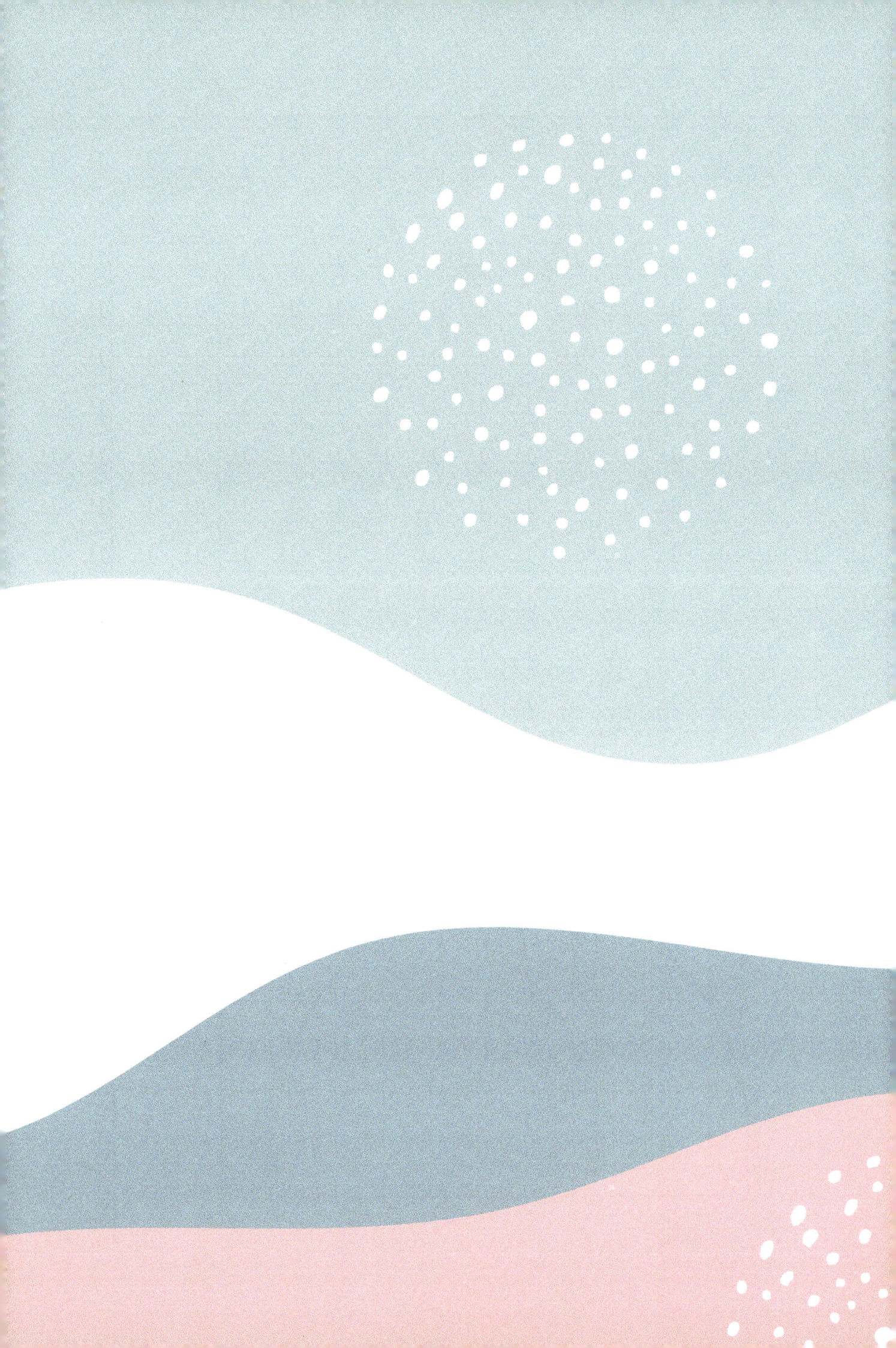

DIRECT-FEEDING

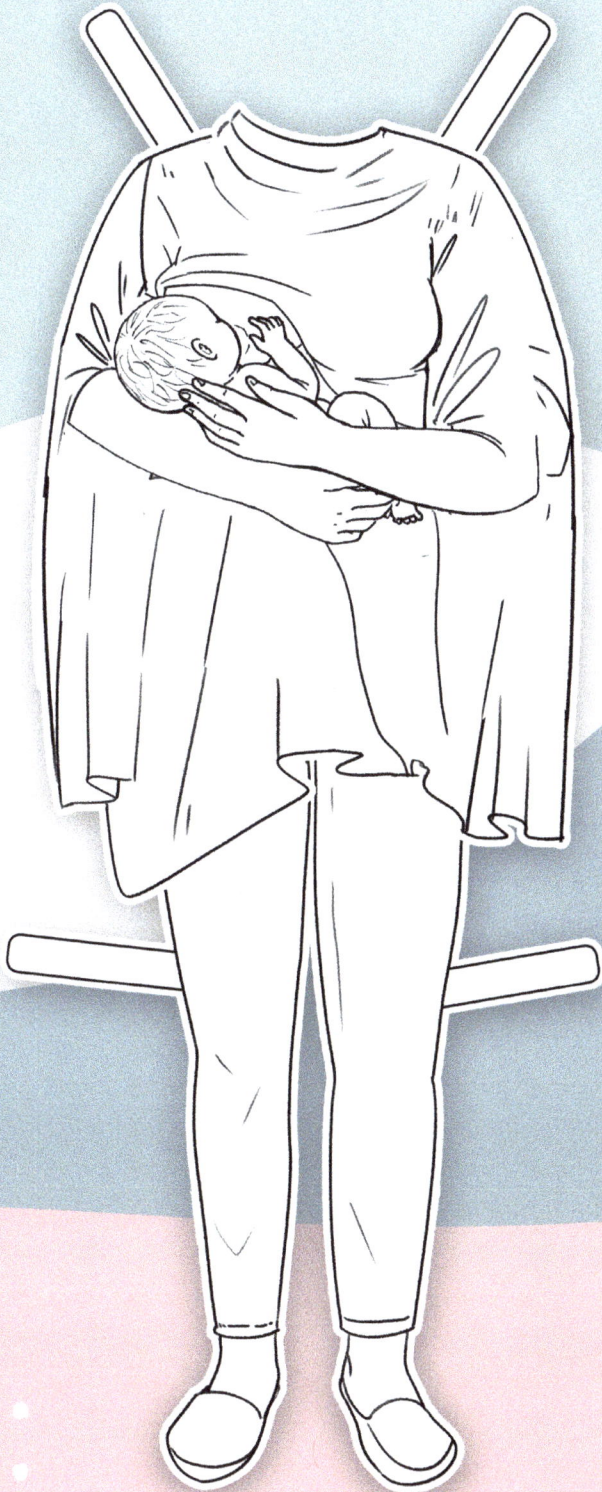

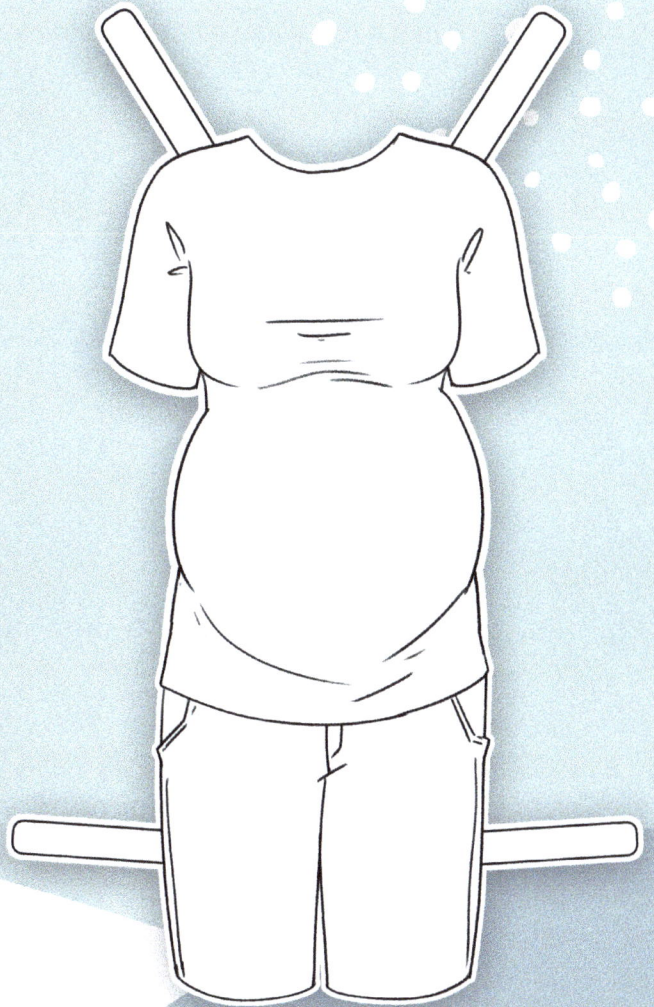

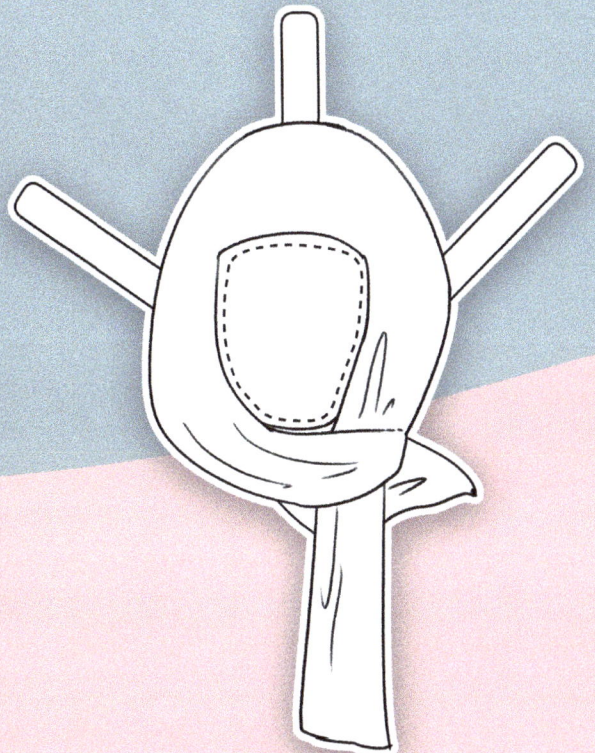

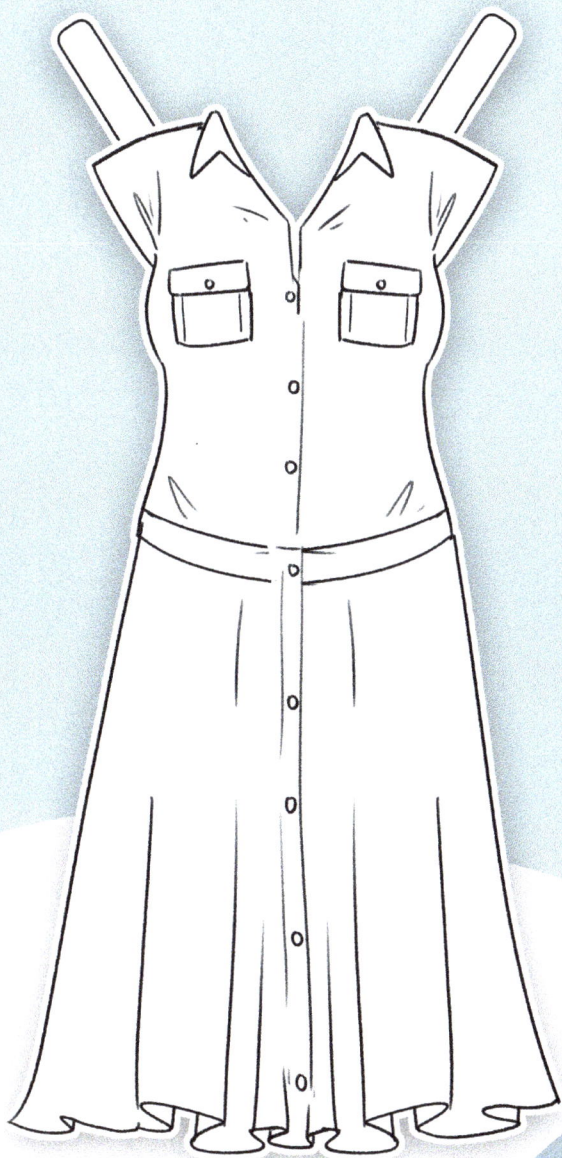

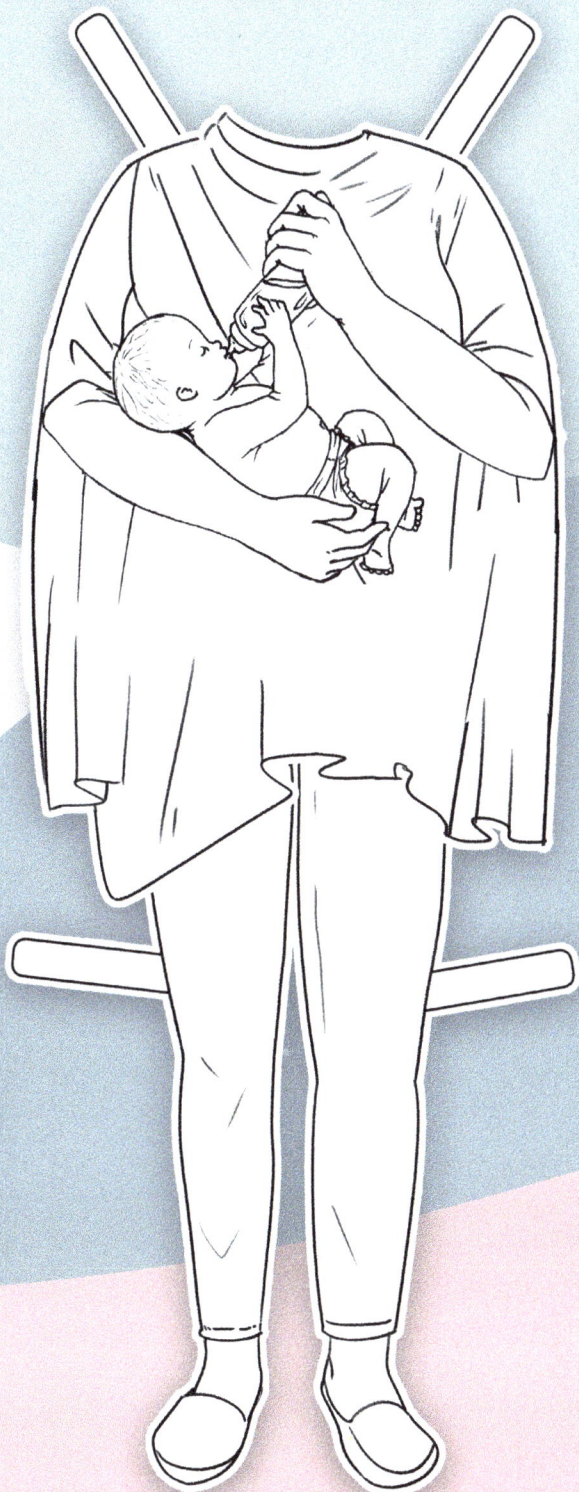

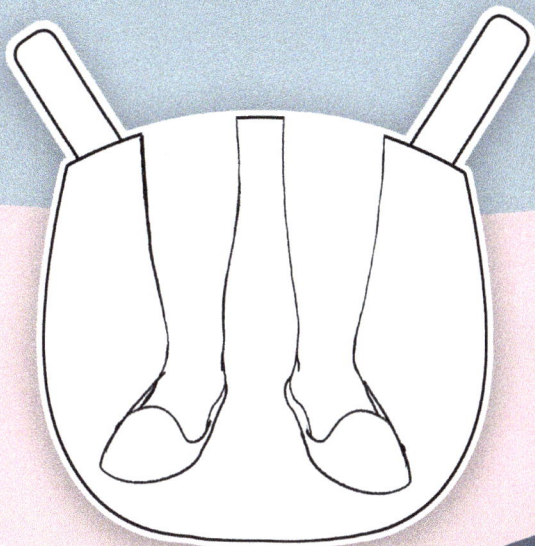

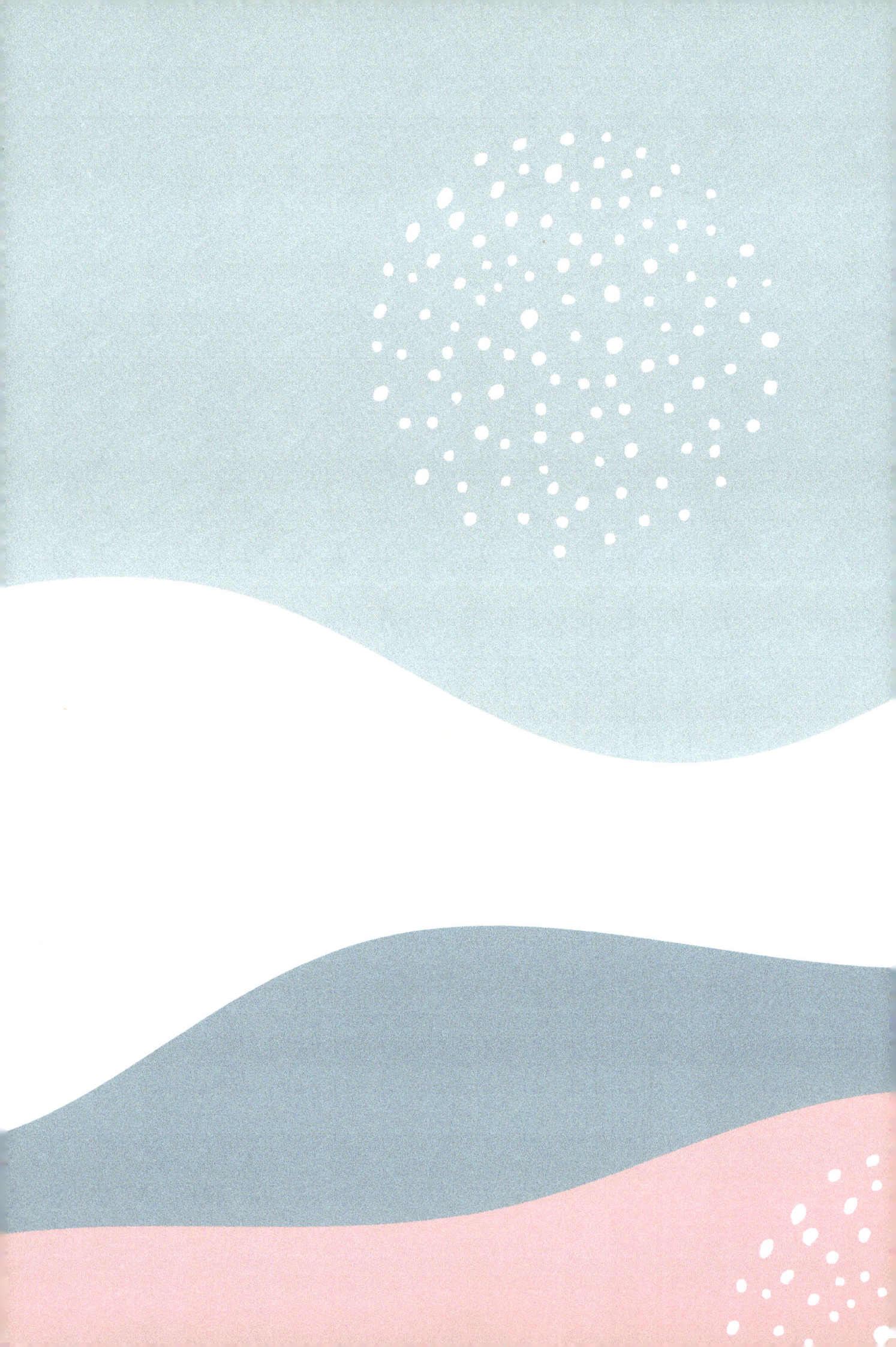

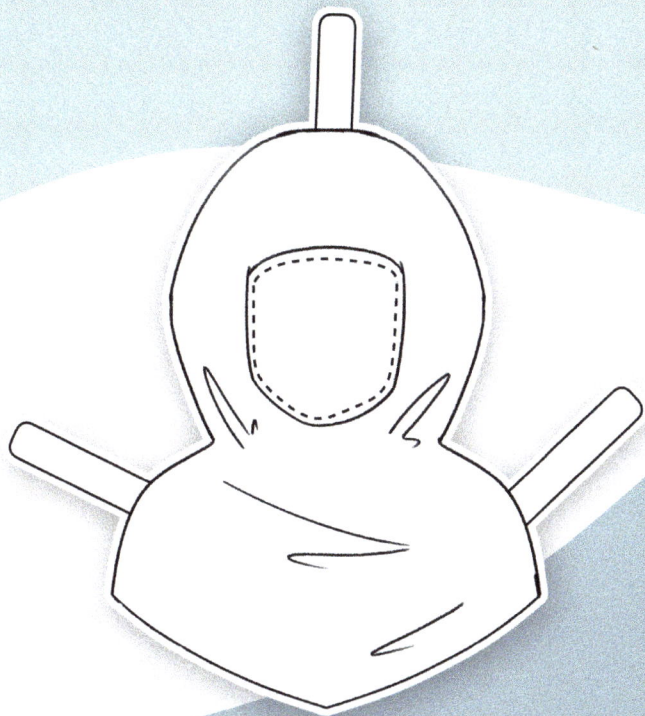

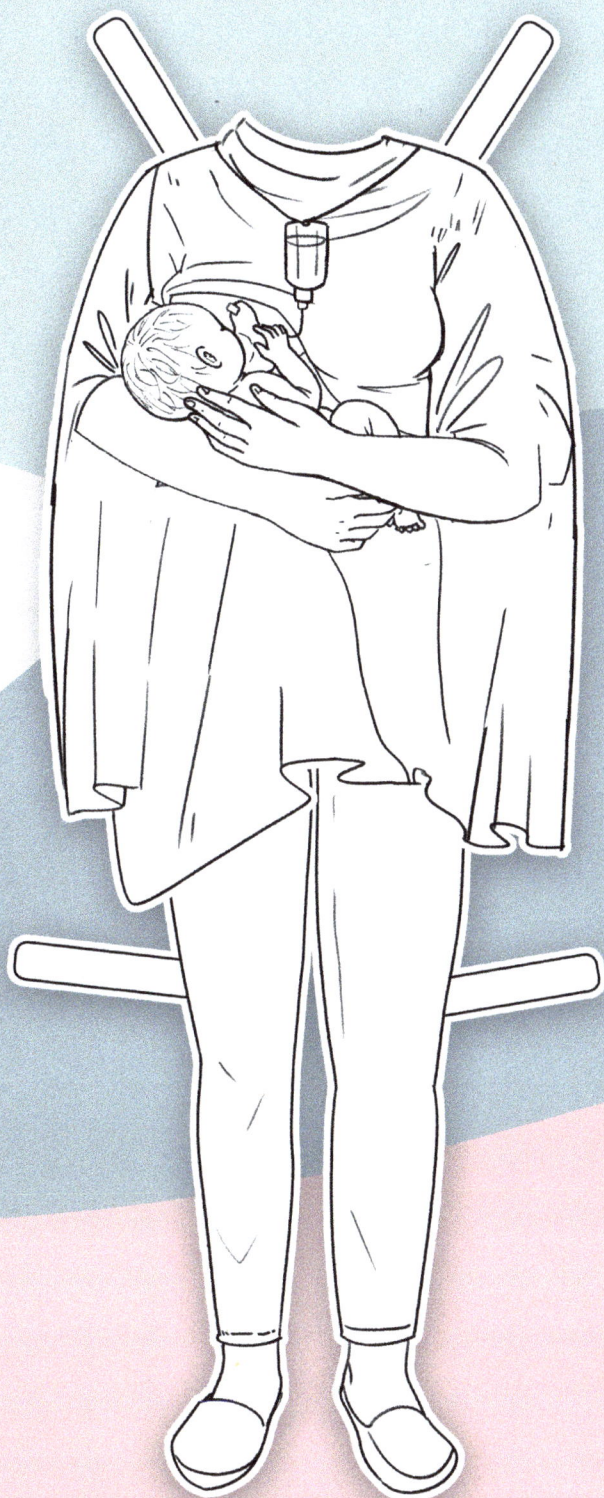

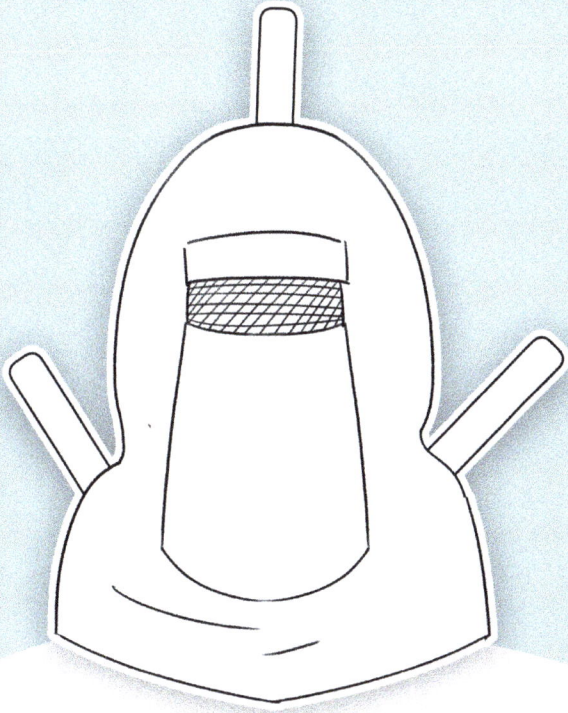

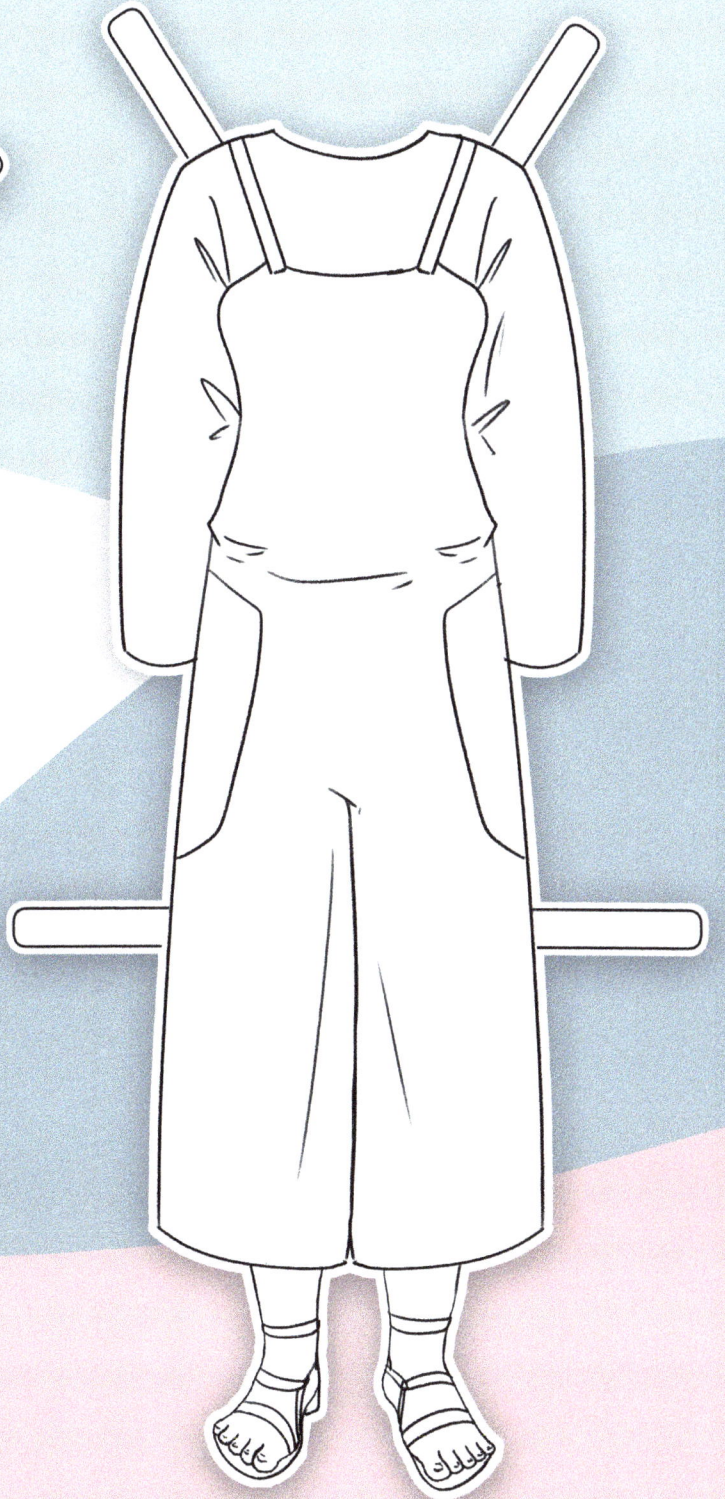

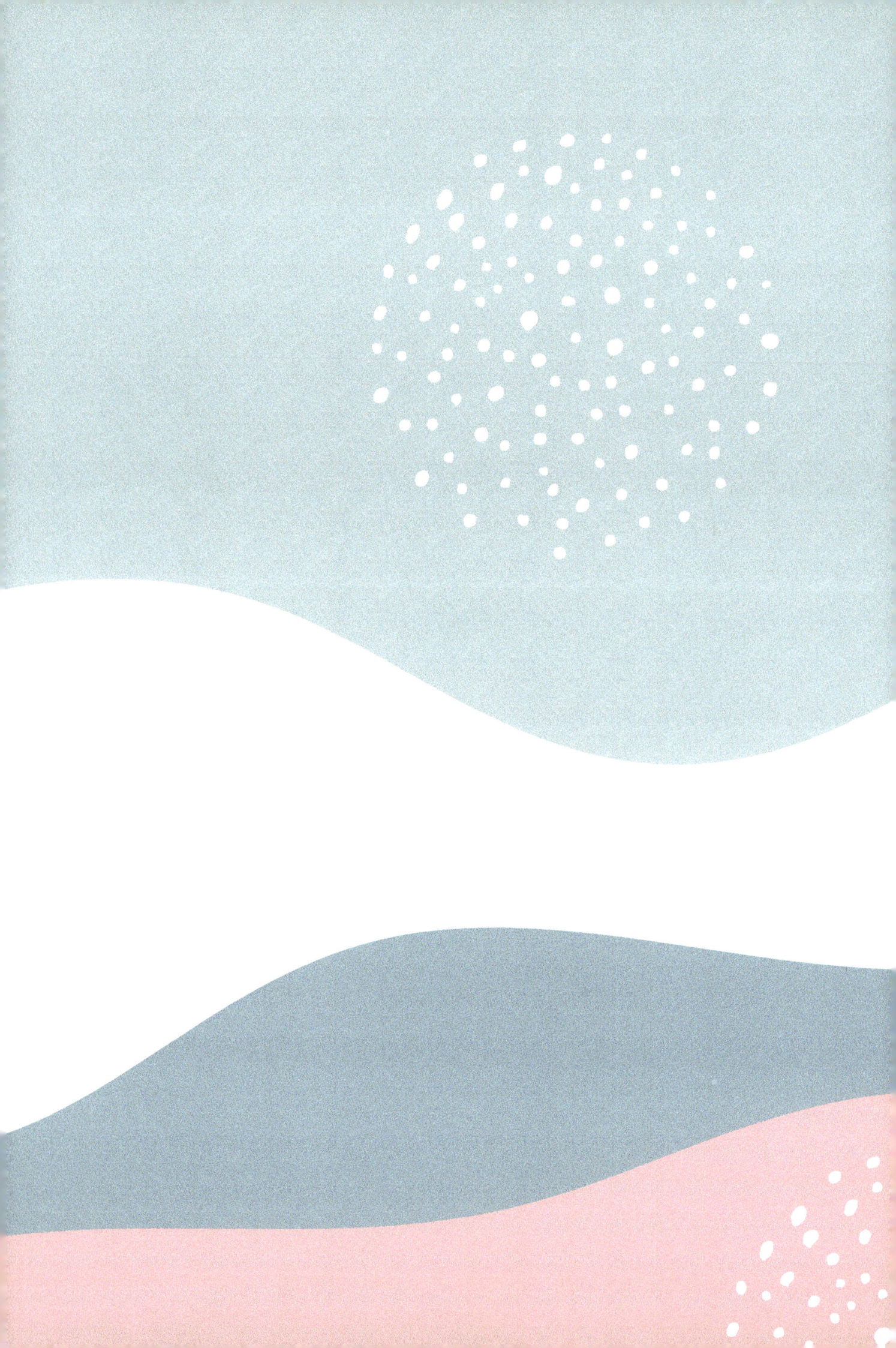

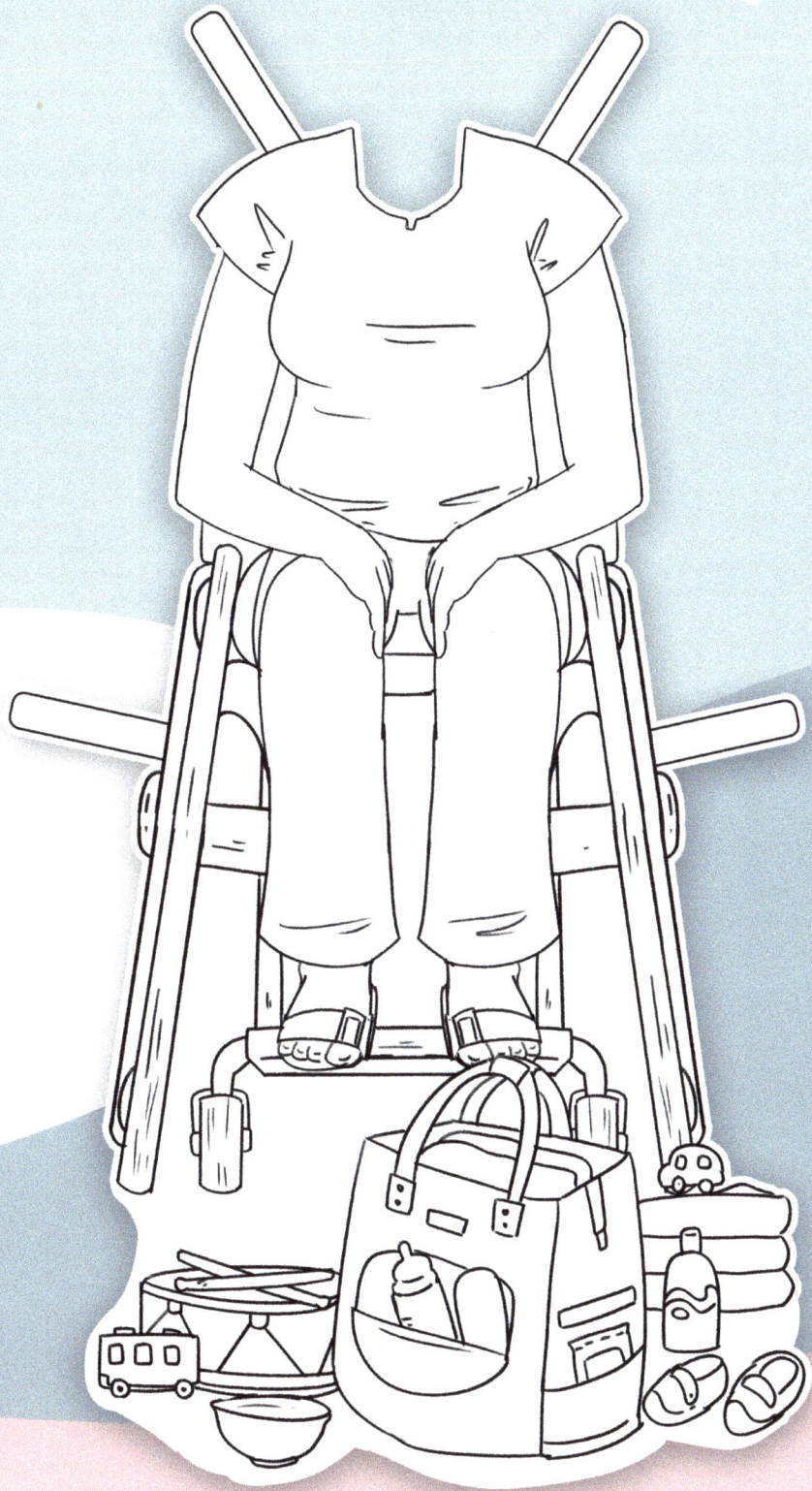

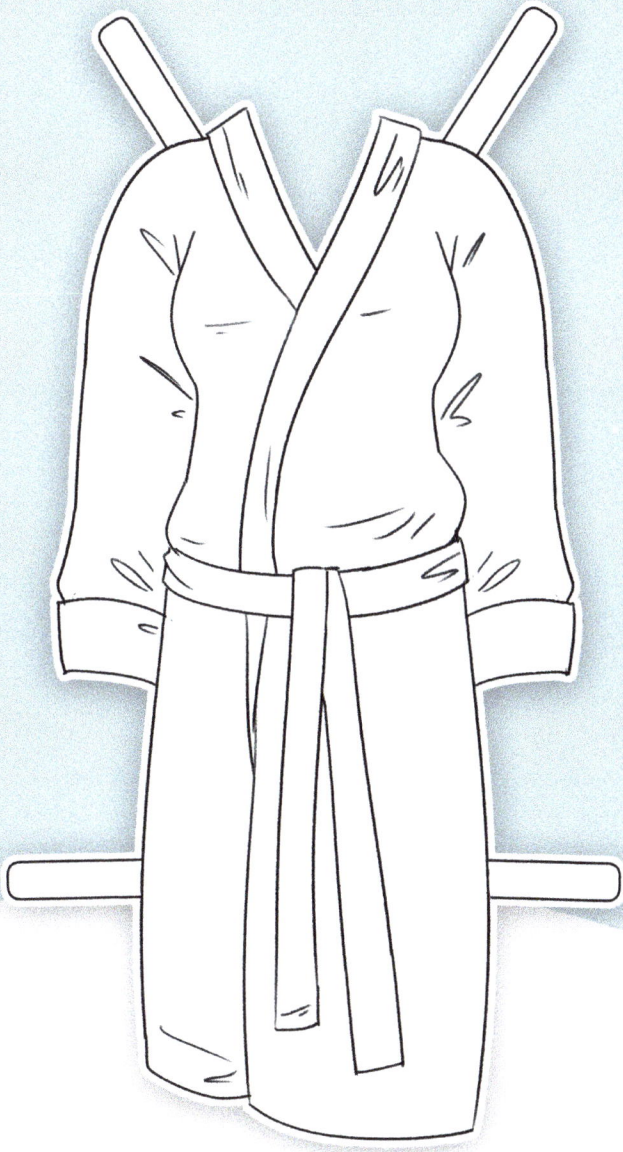

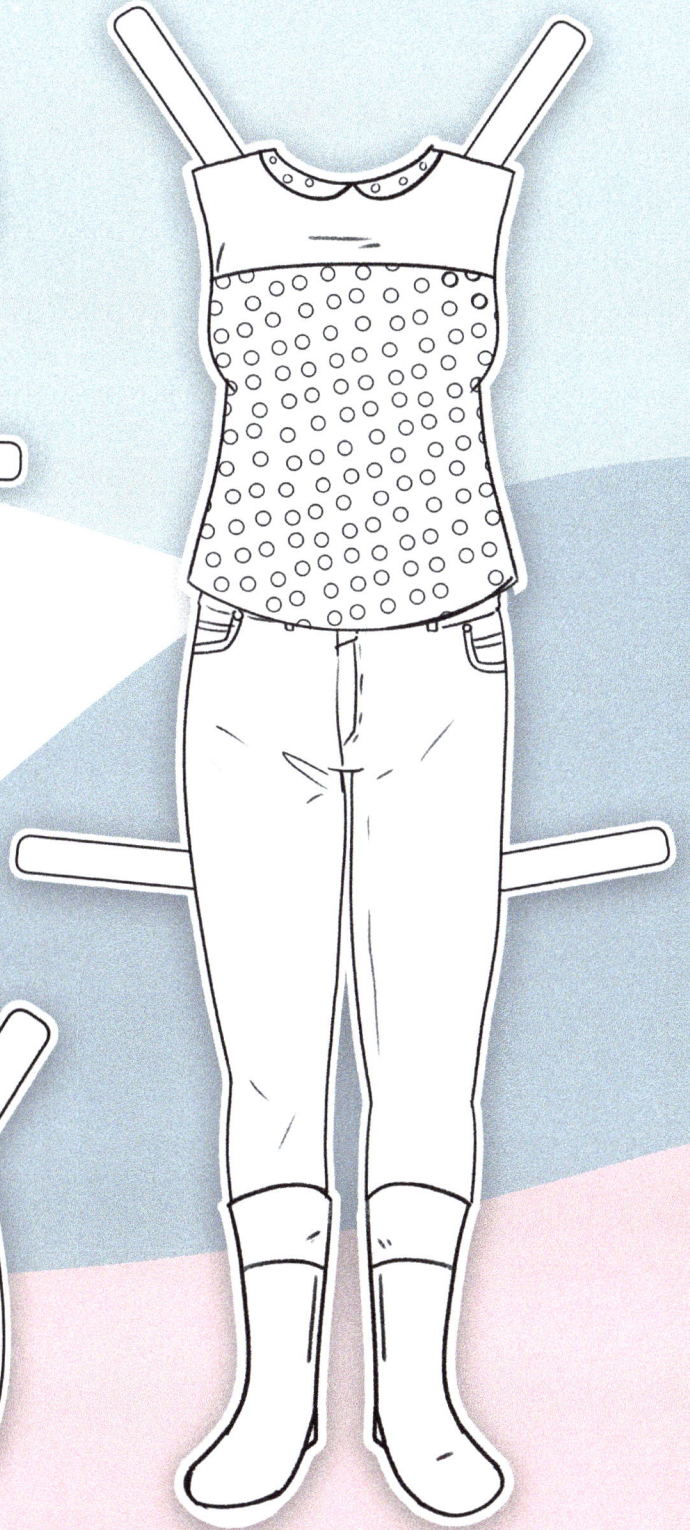

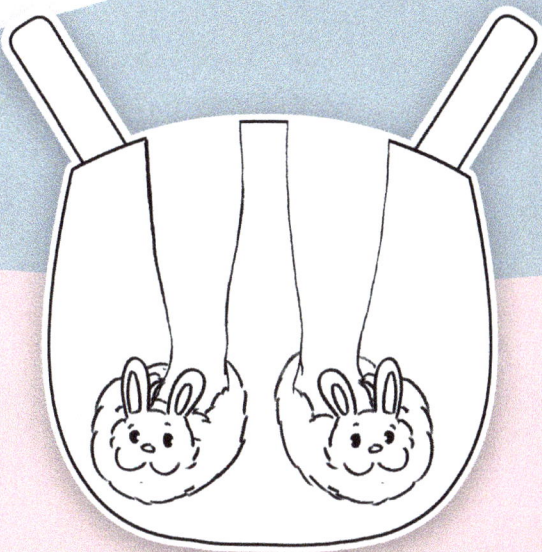

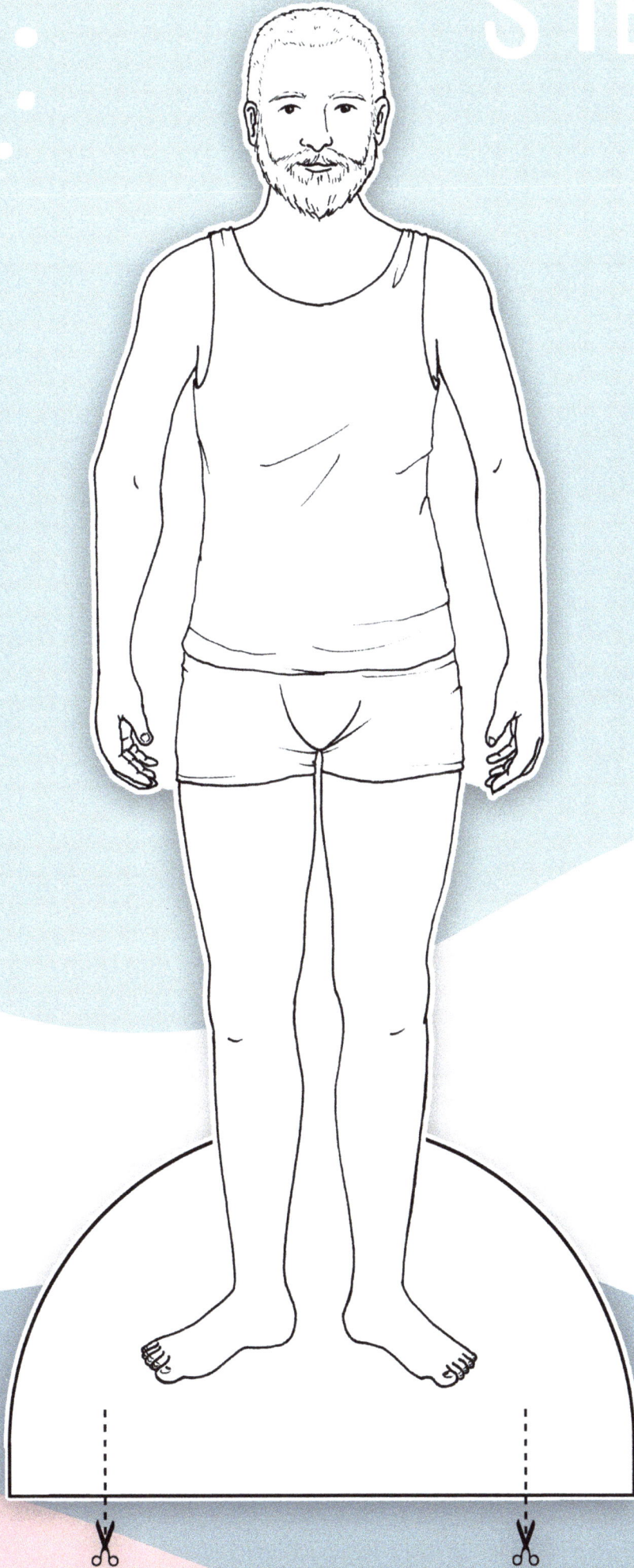

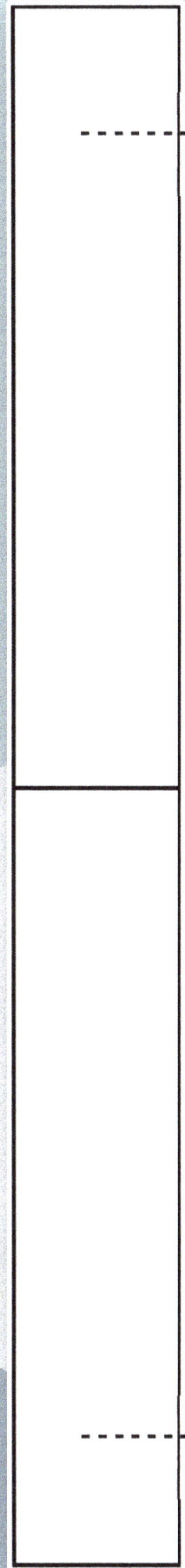

STEVIE

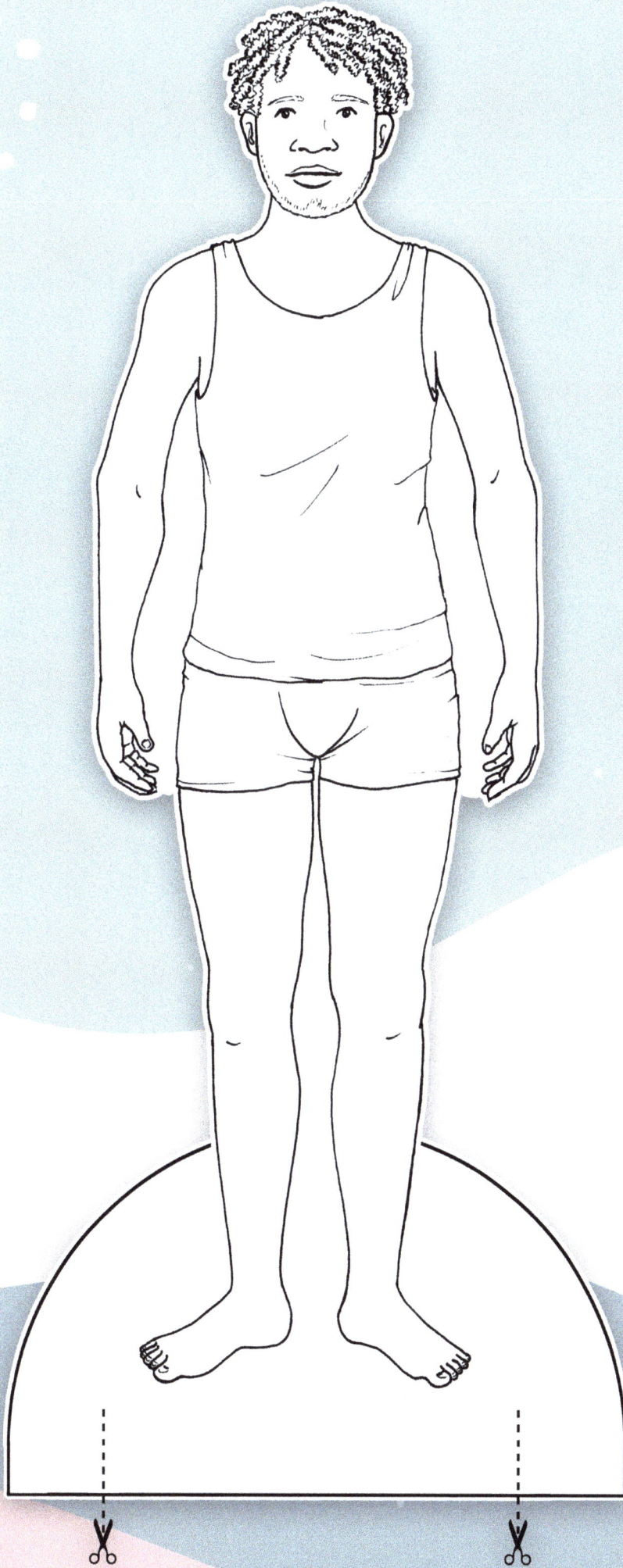

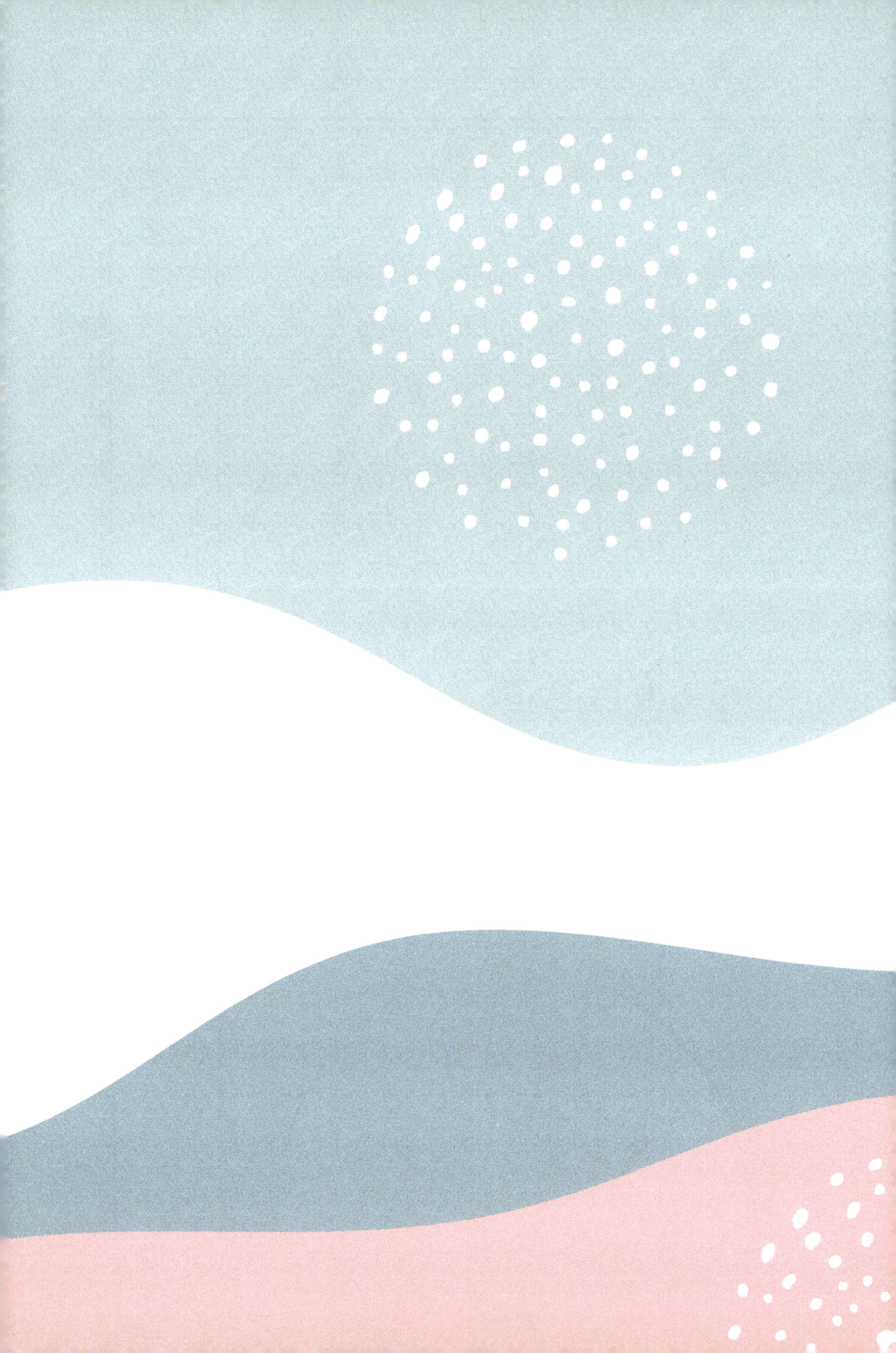

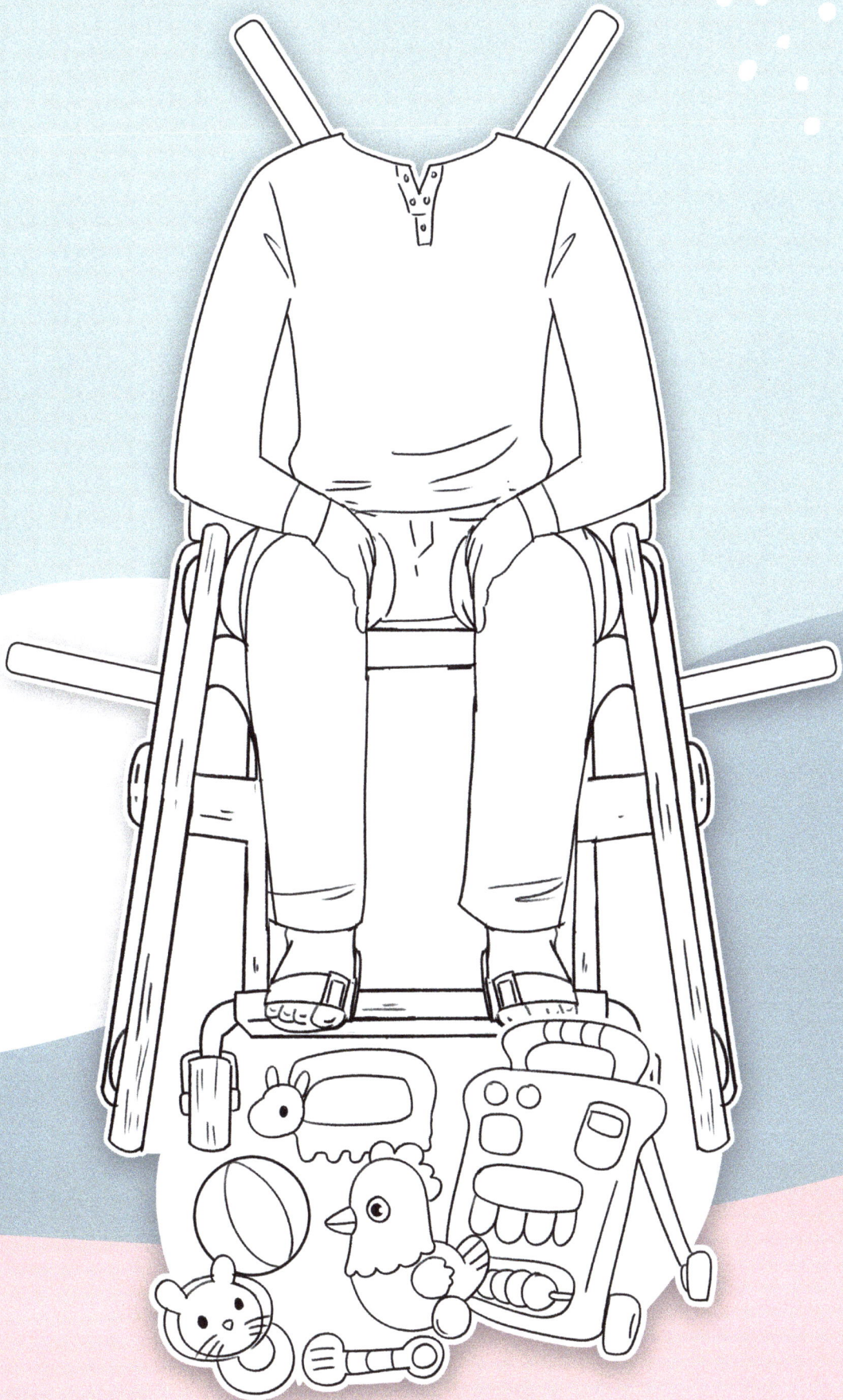

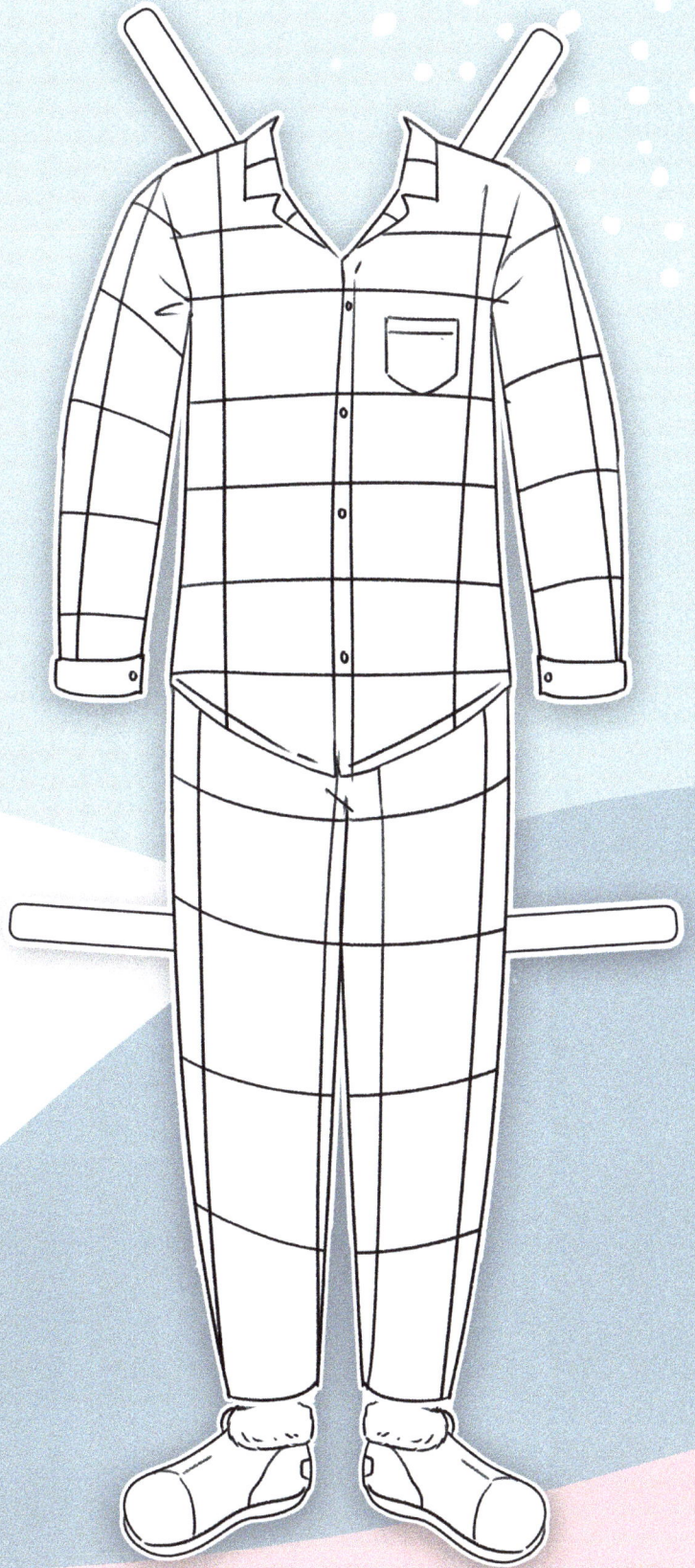

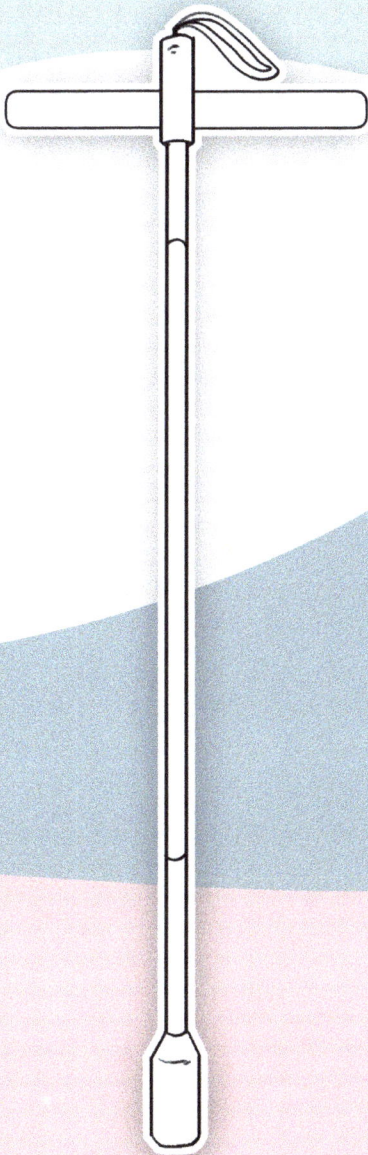

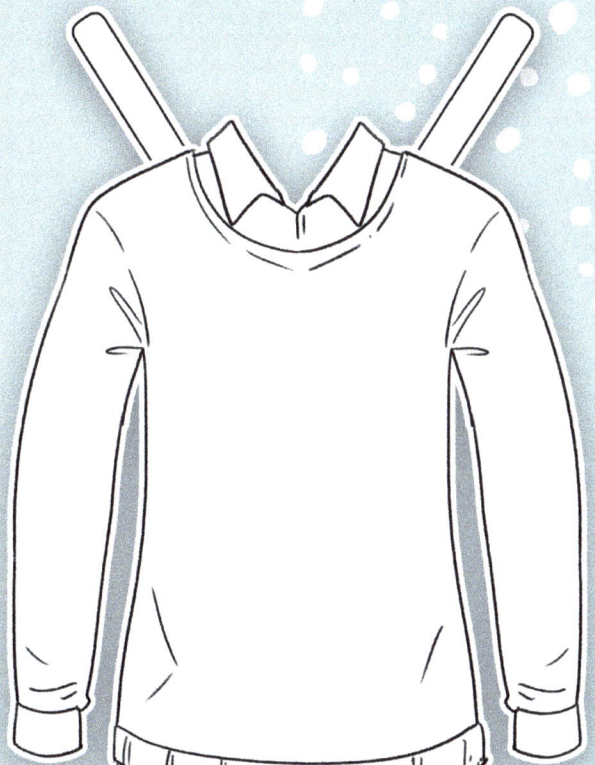

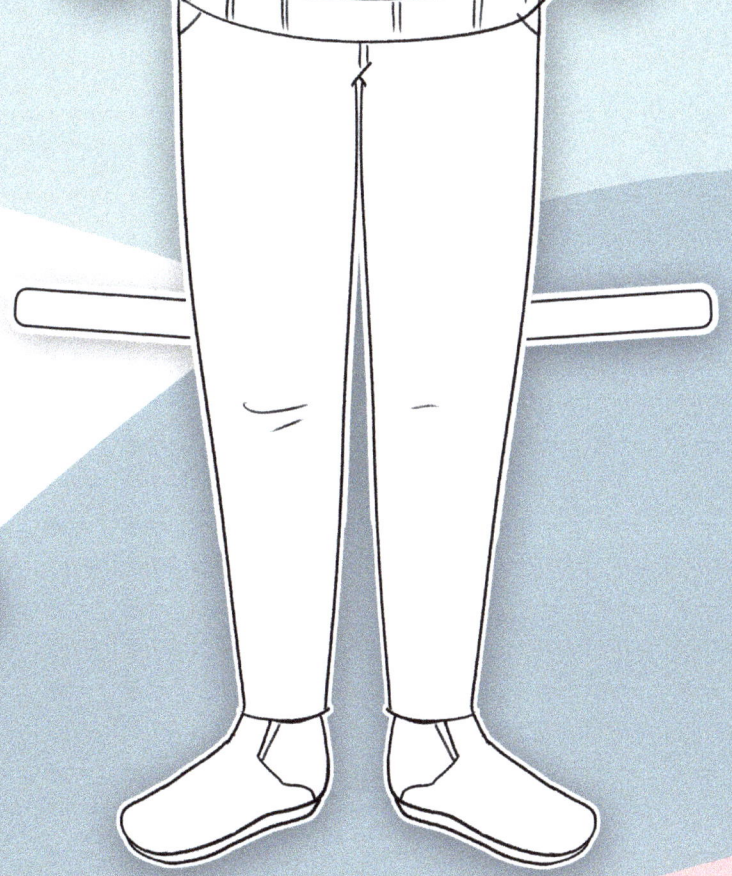

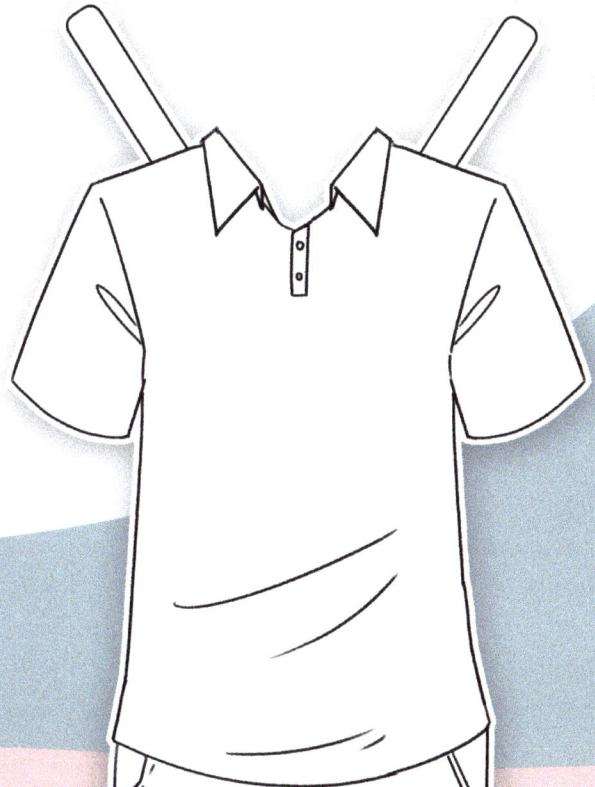

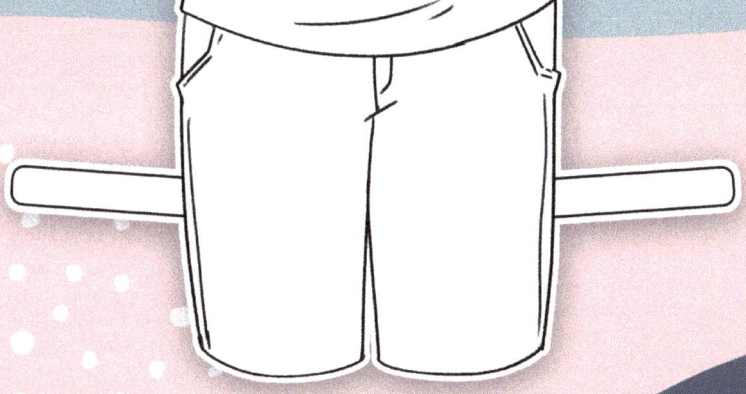

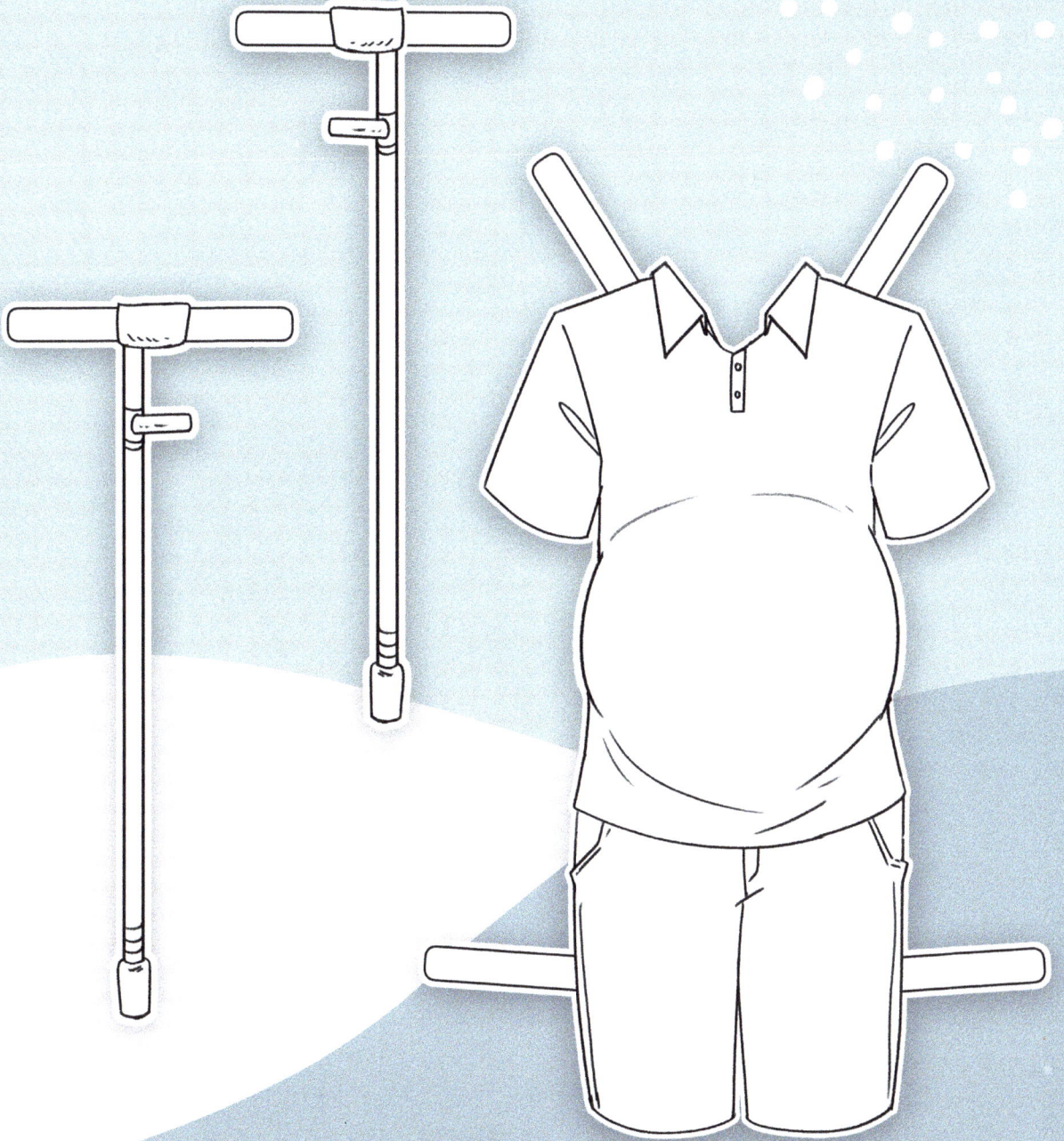

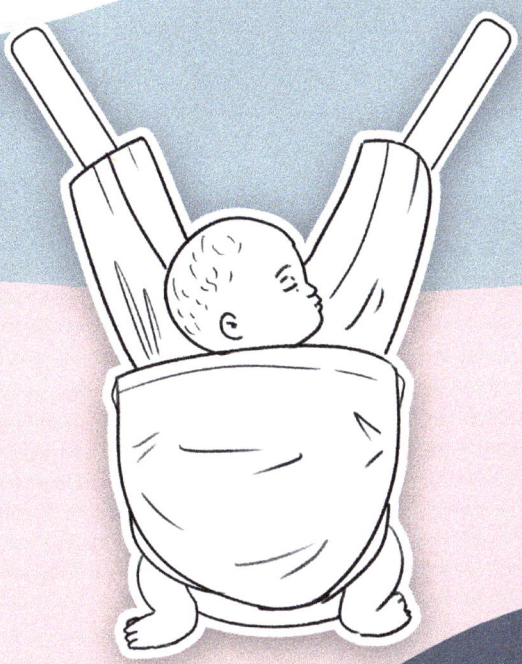

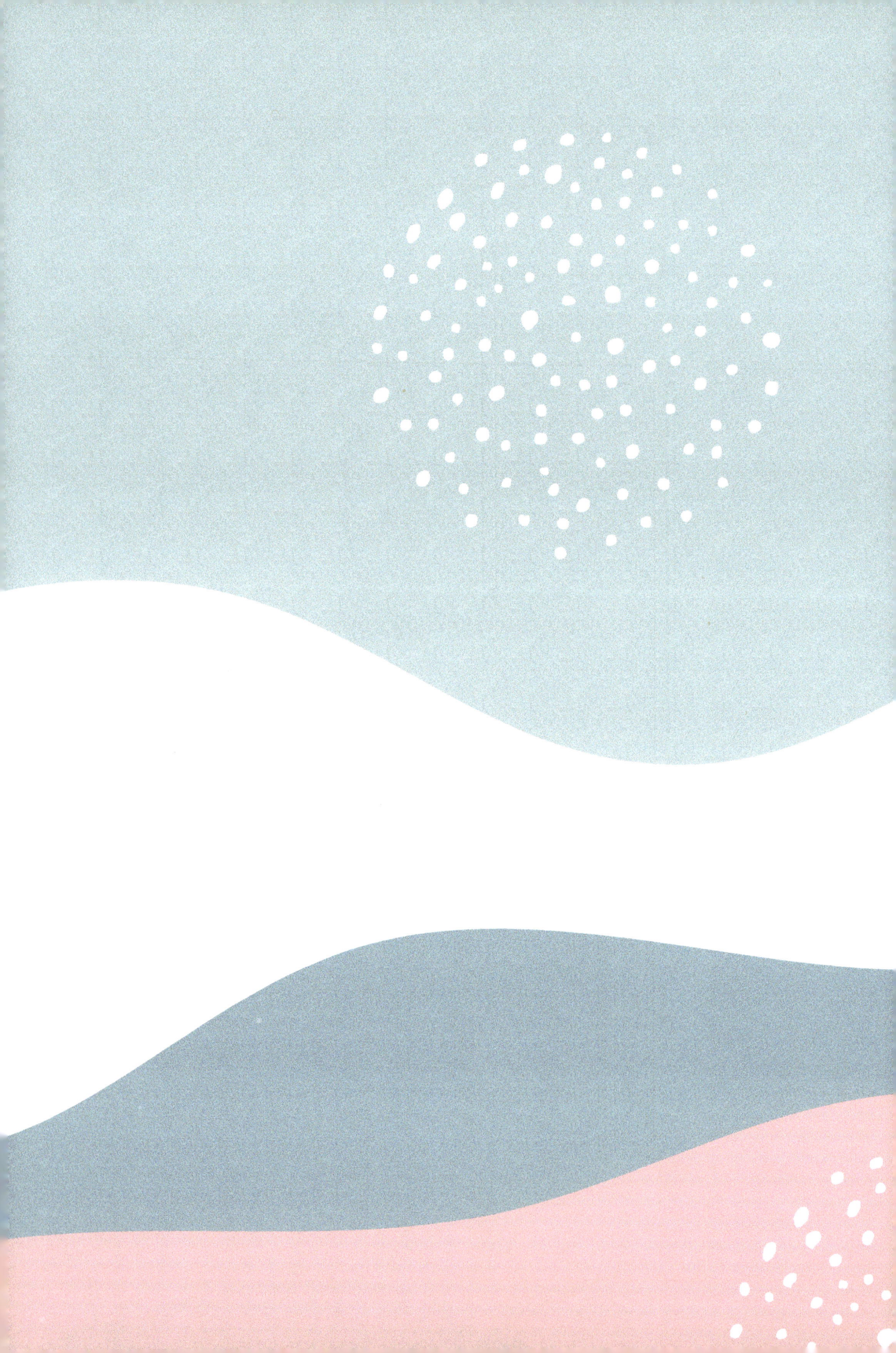

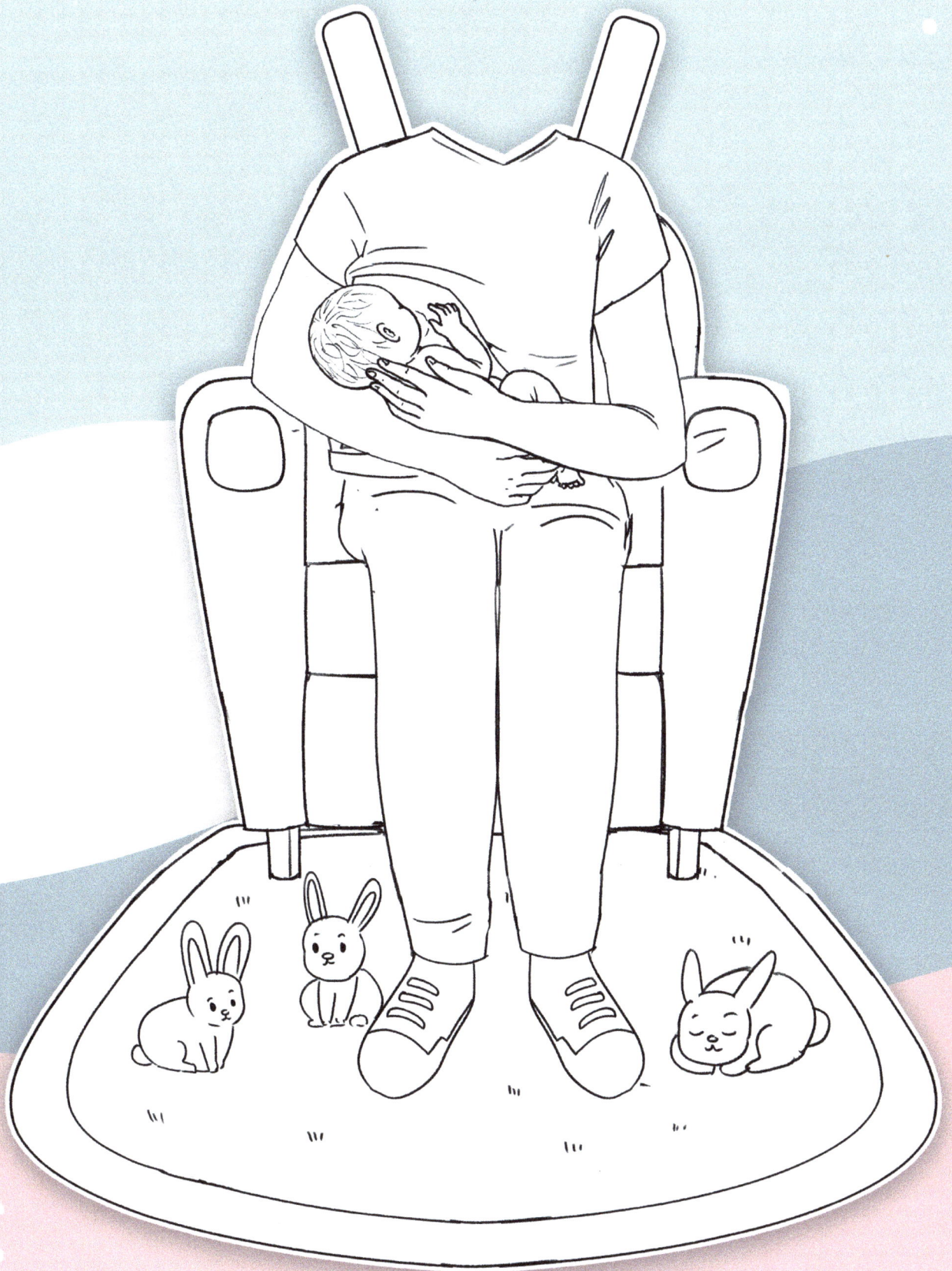

DIRECT-
FEEDING

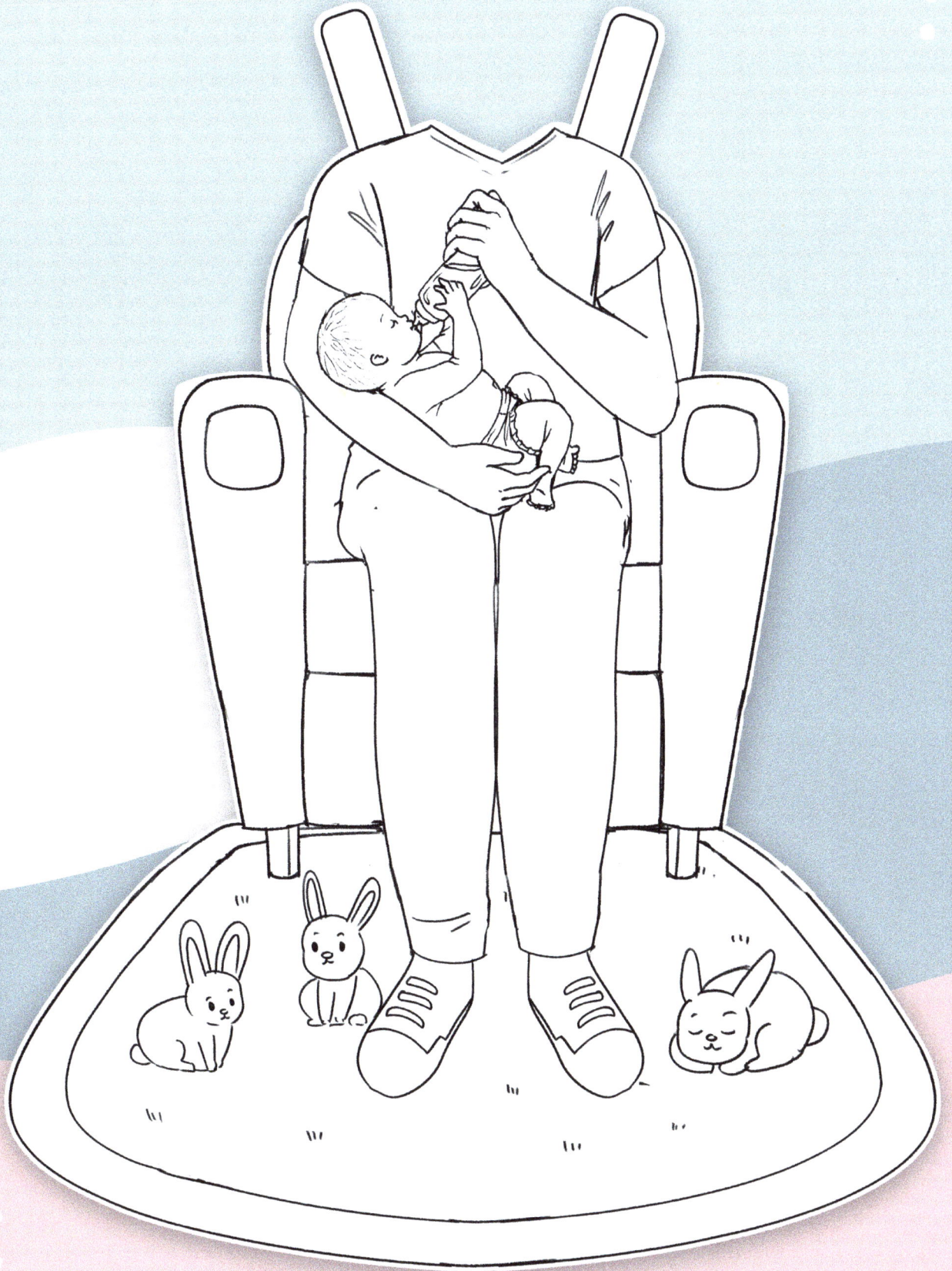

BOTTLE-
FEEDING

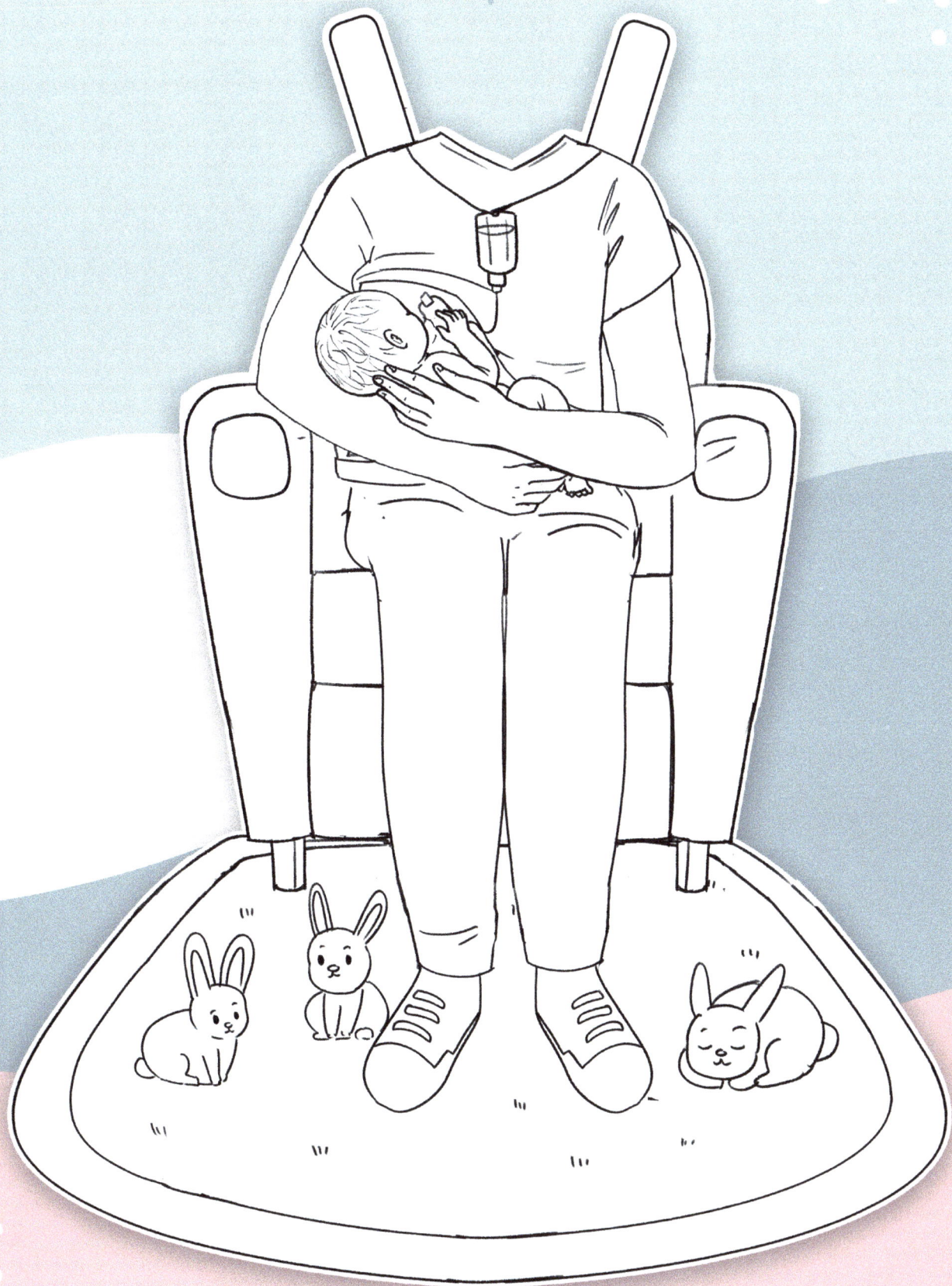

TUBE-
FEEDING

# NOTES TO THE READER

These PaperDolls are the perfect resource to facilitate open and honest conversations with your child about pregnancy and the question of how babies are made. Of course, you may still have some reservations and questions regarding these conversations, such as …

**Aren't they too young to know this?** When kids first ask questions about where babies come from, it isn't sex they're wanting to know about; rather, they're trying to understand where they came from and how they came to exist. Don't feel like you need to rush into explaining sex just yet!

**What if they repeat what I tell them?** Some kids may want to share this information, but you can always ask them not to. Tell them that some parents like to talk to their own kids about where babies come from, and would prefer their children to hear it from them first.

**Won't talking encourage or increase their curiosity?** No, it won't. Talking satisfies curiosity, which means your kids won't have any unanswered questions swimming around their heads.

**Will these conversations worry or scare my child?** Kids are very hard to startle, and they're very good at taking new information in their stride. They're not interested in sex; they just want to understand how babies are made. Plus you'll be giving them information that is age-appropriate.

**Won't this take away their innocence?** No, information empowers your child to make smart decisions about their own bodies. Information isn't harmful and children with this knowledge are no less innocent than those without.

**I find it too embarrassing.** Many parents feel the same. The solution? Start talking when your hands are busy cutting and colouring so you can avoid eye contact with your child. Once you've started, you'll find the conversation gets more relaxed and that subsequent conversations are much easier to start.

**I don't know what to say.** It's easy to feel unsure when starting something new. To help you out, some ideas about how to start conversations and what to talk about are listed below.

## GETTING STARTED

Grab this book, some cardboard (a cereal or biscuit box works), scissors, a glue stick, colouring-in pencils or pens, and tell your child that you have some PaperDolls for them—but first, they'll need to pick which Dolls they want to play with! Ask your child to have a look at the PaperDolls and pick a baby and two adults to colour in.

Casually ask your child some questions about the PaperDolls as they colour them; for example, the Doll's name, what they like to do, what colour hair will they have, etc. Your child may or may not respond.

Use some of the discussion ideas below to start a conversation while your child is colouring, cutting, and playing. If your child requires further information or explanation, **YOU CAN REFER TO THE ILLUSTRATIONS (1–8)** at the back of the book.

# DiSCUSSiON iDEAS

Here are some ideas to consider before talking to your child. Bring these up in conversation to work out how much your child already knows, what they've understood, and whether they need more information. Using the illustrations at the back of the book as a visual aid, start a question-and-answer session with your child, using the simple answers provided below to help them understand.

## CORRECT NAMES OF THE GENITALS

Grab two baby PaperDolls, one with a penis and one with a vulva, and, while pointing out the different body parts, ask your child to name them. Tell your child the correct names for the genitals. These parts include the penis, scrotum, testicle (squishy bit inside the scrotum), vulva, vagina (inside part), and bottom (or anus).

**REFER TO ILLUSTRATION 1.** Point out and name the different body parts for your child.

## THE DIFFERENCE BETWEEN BOYS AND GIRLS

Grab two baby PaperDolls, one with a penis and one with a vulva. Then, point to one and ask your child, 'Is this baby a boy or girl?' Listen to their answer and ask them to explain how they know this. They will probably say that boys have a penis and girls have a vulva.

Explain to your child that, when a baby is born with a penis, everyone will think that the baby is a boy and, when a baby is born with a vulva, everyone will think they are a girl. And most times they are correct. But sometimes they aren't.

When a person with a penis sees themselves as a girl, they are a transgender girl, and when a person with a vulva sees themselves as a boy, they are a transgender boy.

Some children might feel like a mix of boy and girl, or not feel like a boy or girl at all. They are non-binary.

Remind your child that everyone is different and that that's okay.

## WHERE BABIES COME FROM

Ask your child, 'Where do you think babies come from?' Listen to their response and correct any misinformation.

Then, grab an adult PaperDoll (Jo or Lou) and dress it in the pregnant costume. Show it to your child and explain that the Doll is pregnant and that a baby is growing inside them.

Ask your child, 'Where do you think the baby is growing?' They will probably say it grows in the stomach/tummy/belly.

**REFER TO ILLUSTRATION 2.** Point to the uterus and explain that the baby doesn't grow in the stomach; rather, it grows in a special 'baby bag' that is near the stomach. This special place is called the uterus, and is where all babies grow.

## HOW A BABY IS MADE

Grab two adult PaperDolls (Jo or Lou and Stevie or Nick) and one baby PaperDoll. Ask your child, 'Do you know how a baby is made?'

If they say yes, ask them to explain how, and correct any misinformation.

Explain that you need three things to make a baby: a uterus (which is where the baby will grow), a sperm and an egg (which need to join together for the baby to start growing). Explain that the egg usually comes from the person with ovaries and sperm usually comes from the person with testicles.

**REFER TO ILLUSTRATION 3.** Show your child what a sperm and egg look like. You can also explain that they need a uterus, which is where the baby will grow. Point to the joined egg and sperm and explain that, when they join together, a baby will start to grow.

If they want to know where the sperm and egg live, you can explain that the eggs are stored in a special place inside the body called an ovary. The sperm is made inside the body in a place called a testicle.

**REFER TO ILLUSTRATION 4.** Point to the internal organs and show your child the places in which the egg and sperm are found.

# TRANS MAN & NON-BINARY PREGNANCY

*All you need to make a baby is a sperm, an egg and a place to grow the baby (the uterus). This means that a trans man and non-binary person, one of whom has a uterus, are able to become pregnant and give birth to a baby. Children are quite capable of understanding this, especially if reminded of the three things you need to make a baby.*

Grab an adult PaperDoll (Stevie or Nick) and dress them in the pregnant costume. Ask your child, 'Can a man have a baby?' Listen to their response and correct any misinformation.

Explain to your child that you need a uterus to grow a baby, which is something that a female, woman, trans man, or non-binary person may have.

A trans man is a person who was born with a vulva and uterus who identifies as a man/boy (not a woman/girl). They might change their body so that they look more like a man/boy (instead of a woman/girl), but they still have a uterus. This means they can become pregnant and give birth to a baby.

A non-binary person is someone who doesn't identify as either a man/boy or a woman/girl. They might identify as both, neither or something else. If they have a uterus, they can become pregnant and give birth to a baby.

## HOW BABIES GROW

Grab an adult PaperDoll (Jo or Lou) and dress it in the pregnant costume. Point out the pregnant abdomen to your child and ask, 'Have you ever wondered what a baby looks like as it grows inside the uterus?'

**TURN TO ILLUSTRATION 3** and show your child the different stages of foetal development. Explain to your child that the baby starts off very small and that it takes nine months for it to grow fully.

## HOW THE SPERM AND EGG MEET

*Try to not feel overwhelmed by the prospect of this conversation. Kids learn best by being presented with small snippets of information that are then repeated. They'll forget most of what you say and will view sex as just another part of making a baby.*

Your child might request more information—for example, how the sperm gets from one body to another. There are several ways to explain this.

**REFER TO ILLUSTRATION 5** for an explanation that **doesn't mention sexual intercourse**. Point to the relevant illustration and explain that the sperm comes out through the penis and goes into the vagina, which is where it finds the egg.

**REFER TO ILLUSTRATION 6** for an explanation that **includes sexual intercourse**. If they want to know how the sperm gets inside the vagina, you can explain that there are lots of different ways to make a baby. One way is when an adult lets another adult place their penis into their vagina (explain that this process is called 'sex' or 'sexual intercourse').

## ASSISTED REPRODUCTION

Explain to your child(ren) that sometimes people need help to make a baby, which means the sperm and egg might join together in a way that doesn't involve sexual intercourse. The people might need to get sperm or an egg from someone else, in which case a special doctor will help the egg and sperm join together so as to make a baby.

Explain how your child was made (adapt these descriptions to suit your family). You can also use the PaperDolls to help illustrate who was needed.

Start off with, 'We needed some help to make you.' Then, use the following prompts to help.

**Sperm and/or egg donation:** Someone gave us some sperm/eggs, and some special doctors helped join them together.

**Assisted reproduction (IVF/IUI):** A doctor helped to get the sperm and egg to meet, and then they put you in my/your birth mother's uterus, which is where you grew.

**Surrogacy:** We used someone else's uterus to grow you. A special doctor helped to get the sperm and egg to meet, and then put you inside someone with a uterus, which is where you grew.

**Adoption:** The sperm and egg that made you didn't come from us. You were already growing in the uterus of the person who gave birth to you.

**REFER TO ILLUSTRATION 7** to help explain the different ways that reproduction can occur.

## DIFFERENT TYPES OF FAMILIES

Grab a baby and all of the adult PaperDolls. Explain to your child that there are many different family types and that you don't always need a mother and a father to make a baby. Some families have just one parent, while others have two parents of a different sex or the same sex.

Ask your child to show you, using the PaperDolls, what type of family they have.

## HOW BABIES ARE BORN

Grab an adult PaperDoll (Jo or Lou) and dress it in the pregnant costume. Ask your child, 'How do you think a baby gets out of the uterus?' Listen to their response and correct any misinformation.

Explain that babies come out through the vagina or through a special hole cut into the abdomen.

**REFER TO ILLUSTRATION 8** and show your child the ways in which a baby can come out.

## HOW A BABY IS FED

*There are many ways to feed a baby: direct-feeding, bottle-feeding, and tube-feeding, for instance.*

*Parents typically feed their baby in the way that feels best for them.*

*'Direct-feeding' describes the process where a baby is fed directly from their body. A woman, non-binary person, trans man can direct-*

feed. A trans woman may also direct-feed their baby with the support of medications and a pump.

'Tube-feeding' describes the process by which a baby is fed using an 'at-chest supplementer', a device that allows milk to be given while the baby is feeding at the breast or chest. A tube is placed next to the nipple and, when the baby latches onto the nipple, milk will travel from a bottle through the tube as the baby sucks.

Grab two of the adult PaperDolls (Jo or Lou and Stevie or Nic) and all of the feeding costumes.

Ask your child, 'How do you think a baby eats?' After they answer, explain that babies start off by drinking milk, which can come from the breasts (or chest or nipples) or from a baby's bottle.

Ask your child to show you, using the PaperDolls, how a baby might be fed.

Ask your child, 'How do you think a man might feed a baby?' Listen to their response and explain that most men will bottle feed a baby.

To be inclusive of how a transgender or non-binary person can feed their baby, explain that some trans men may direct-feed their baby. If they can't make enough milk for the baby, they can use a supplementer (where a thin tube will carry milk from a bottle to the nipple). Dress Stevie or Nic in the different costumes to illustrate the different ways in which feeding can occur.

# 1 WHAT ARE THE NAMES OF THE DIFFERENT BODY PARTS?

**BABY ASSIGNED FEMALE AT BIRTH**

**BABY ASSIGNED INTERSEX AT BIRTH**

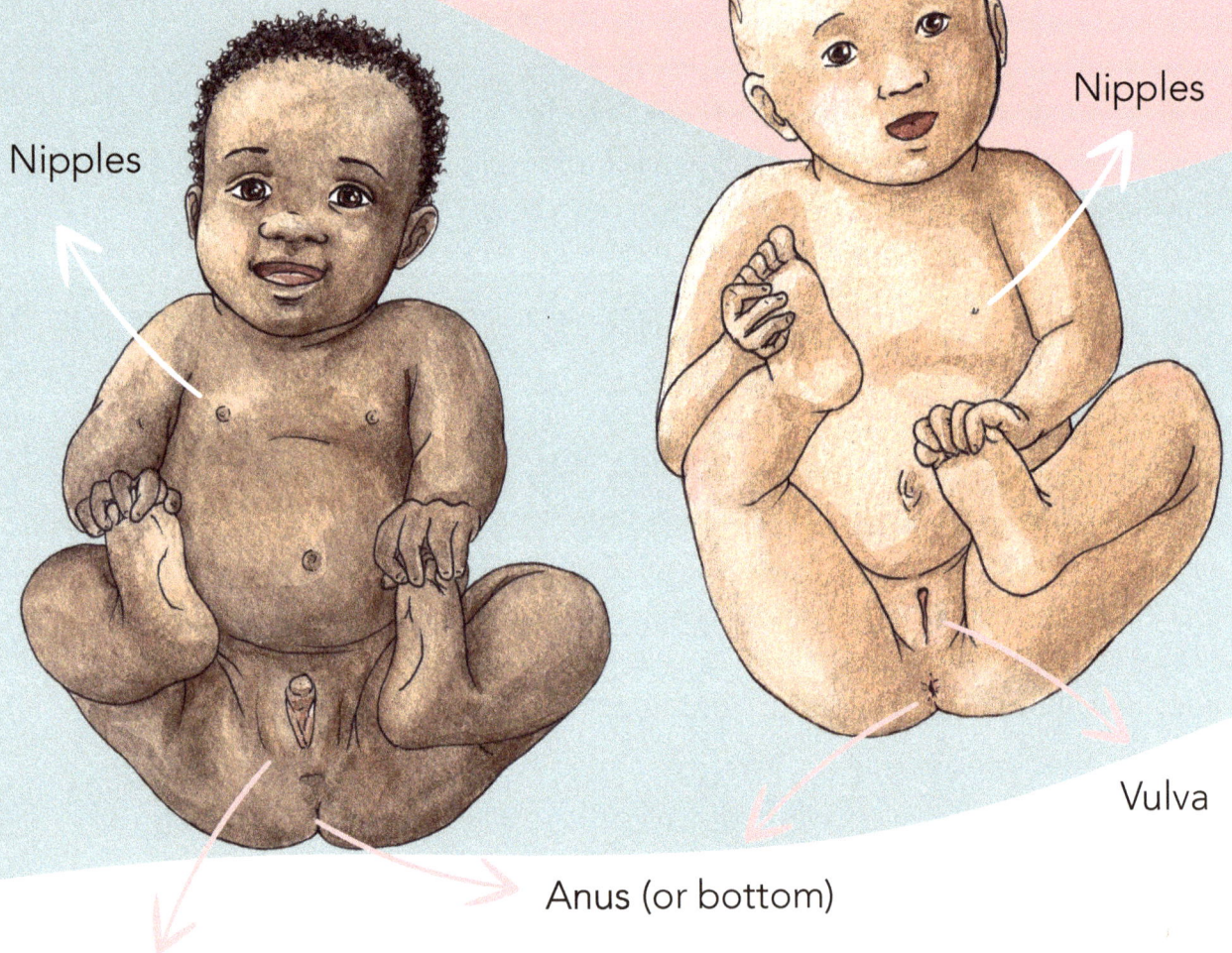

Nipples

Nipples

Vulva

Anus (or bottom)

This baby has genitals that look different to a penis or vulva.

Sometimes a baby is born with genitals that look different. They might look different on the outside and/or the inside of their body. When this happens, the baby is usually assigned intersex at birth.

Sometimes people don't find out that they are intersex until they start to grow up or are fully grown up.

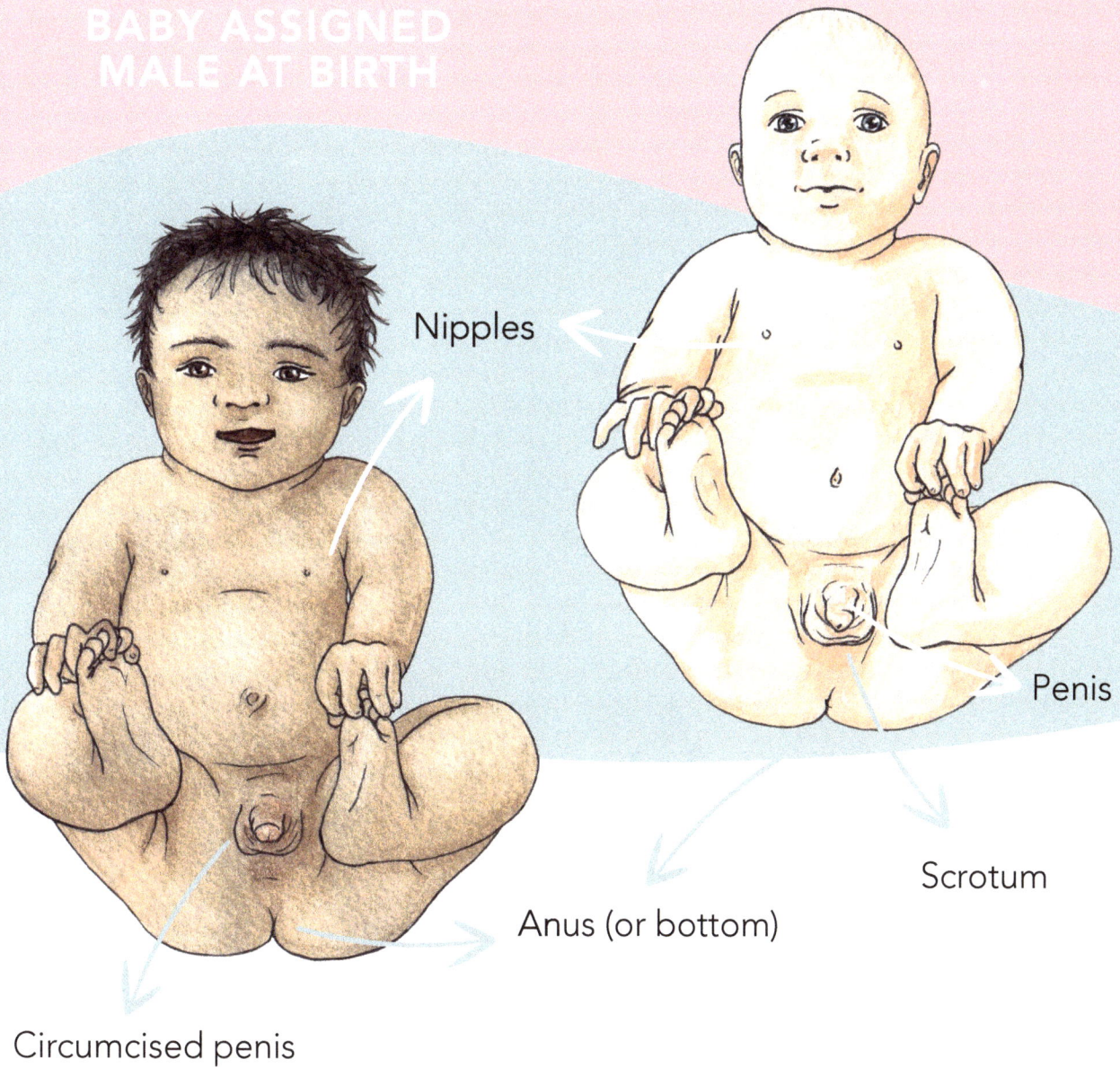

BABY ASSIGNED
MALE AT BIRTH

BABY ASSIGNED
MALE AT BIRTH

Nipples

Penis

Anus (or bottom)

Scrotum

Circumcised penis

Some penises look different because they have the
foreskin removed. This is called circumcision and
it is done for religious or medical reasons. It might
happen when they are a baby, a child or an adult.

# **2** WHERE DOES THE BABY GROW?

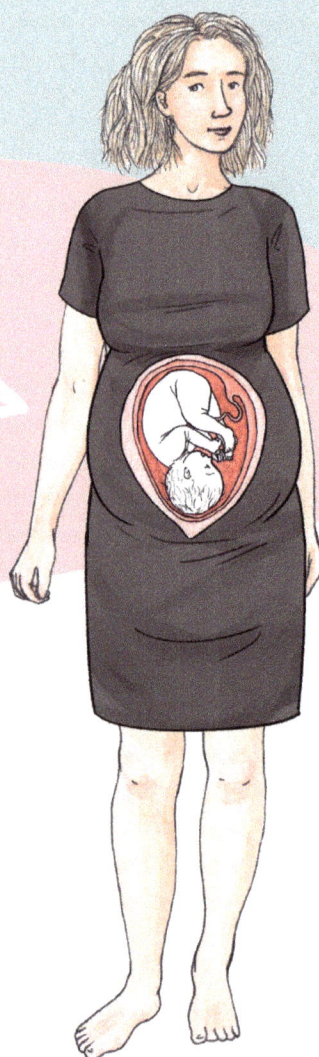

The baby grows
inside the uterus.

## WHAT DOES THE BABY
## LOOK LIKE AS IT GROWS?

The cell will divide into two cells and keep on
dividing until a ball of cells is made.

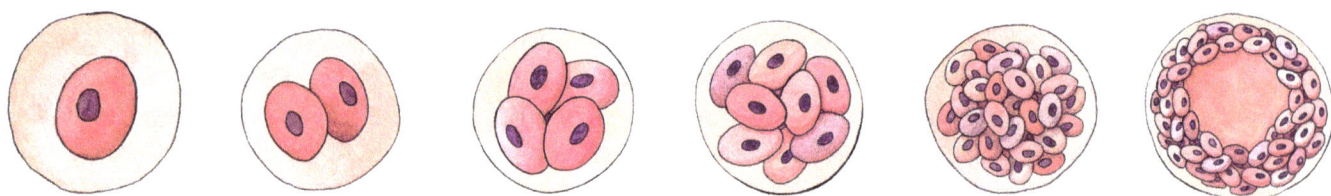

**THE FIRST TWO WEEKS**

The ball will then plant itself inside the uterus. From
there, it will grow and slowly form a baby. It takes
around nine months for the baby to fully grow.

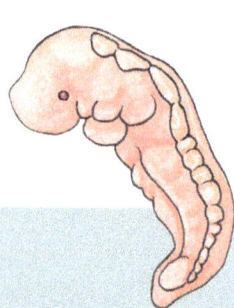  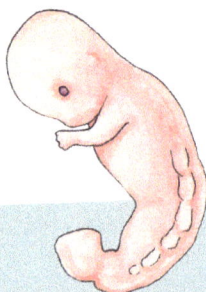  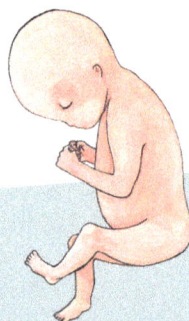  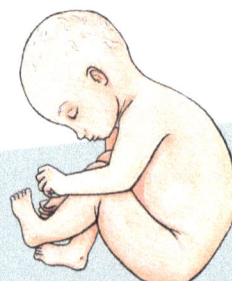

1 MONTH          2 MONTHS          4 MONTHS          9 MONTHS

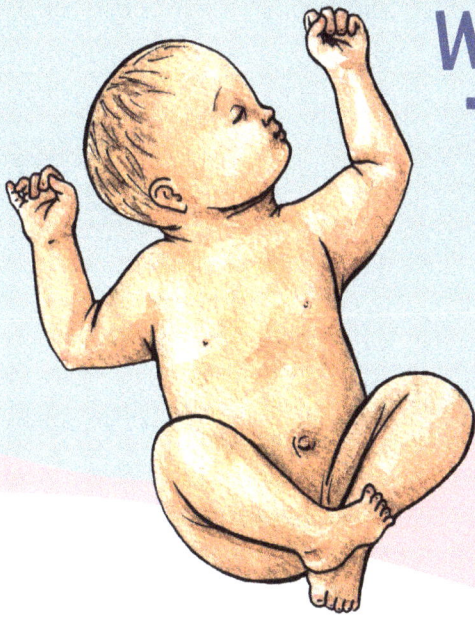

# WHAT DO YOU NEED TO MAKE A BABY?

**3**

You need three things to make a baby. A sperm, an egg and a uterus.

This is what a sperm looks like up close.

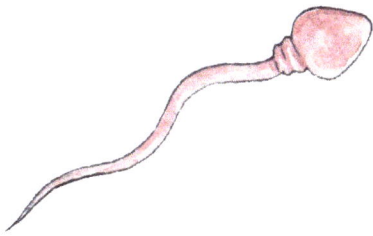

This is what an egg looks like up close.

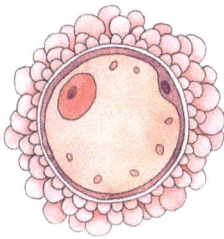

This is what the uterus looks like inside the body.

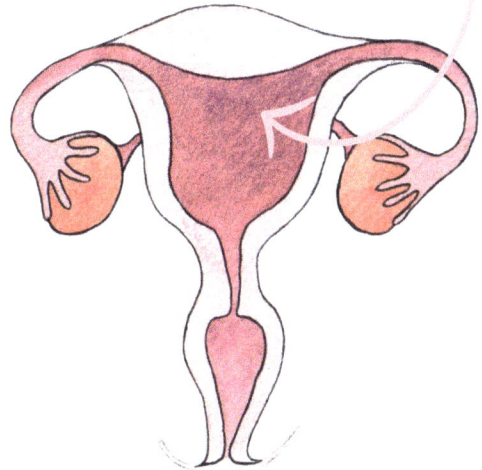

Another name for the egg is ovum.

**A BABY WILL START TO GROW WHEN THE SPERM JOINS WITH AN EGG.**

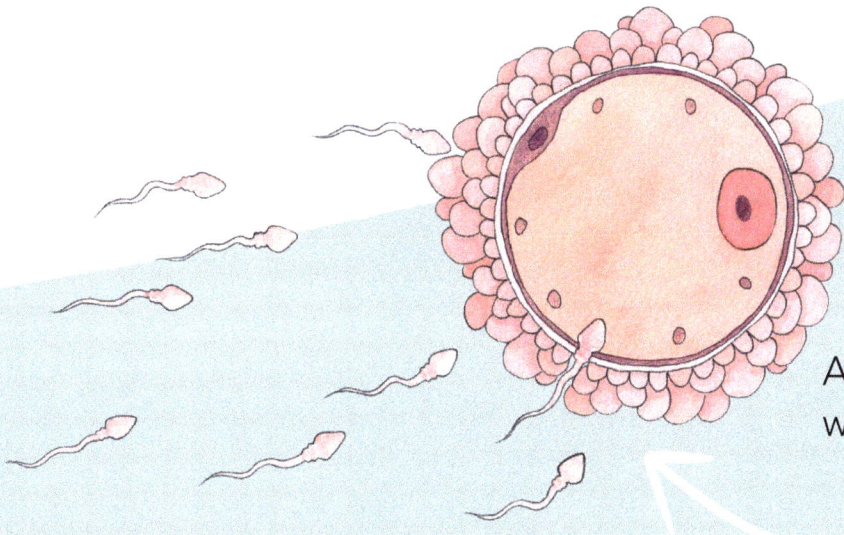

Another name for the uterus is the womb.

A sperm has joined with an egg.

# WHERE DO THE SPERM AND EGG LIVE?

The sperm is so small that you can't see it.

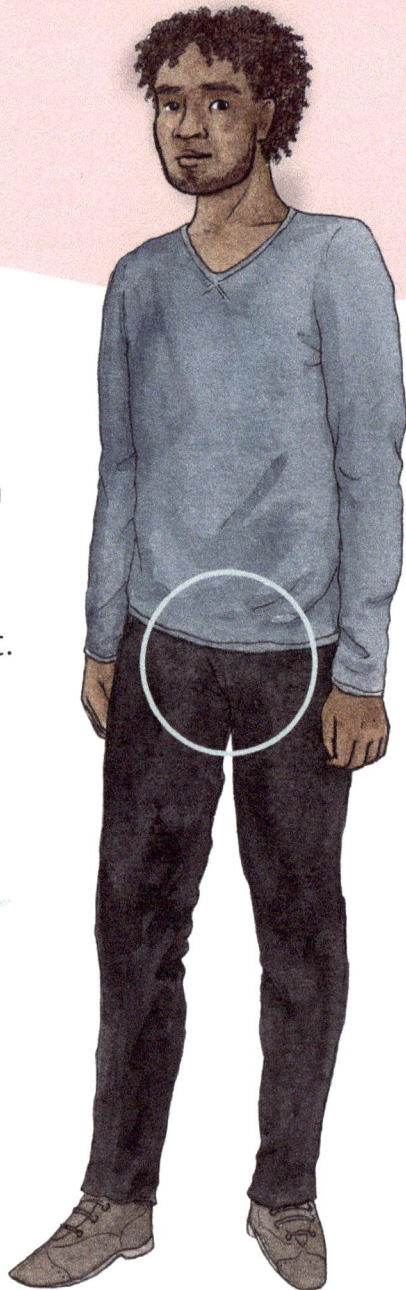

The egg is as small as this dot.

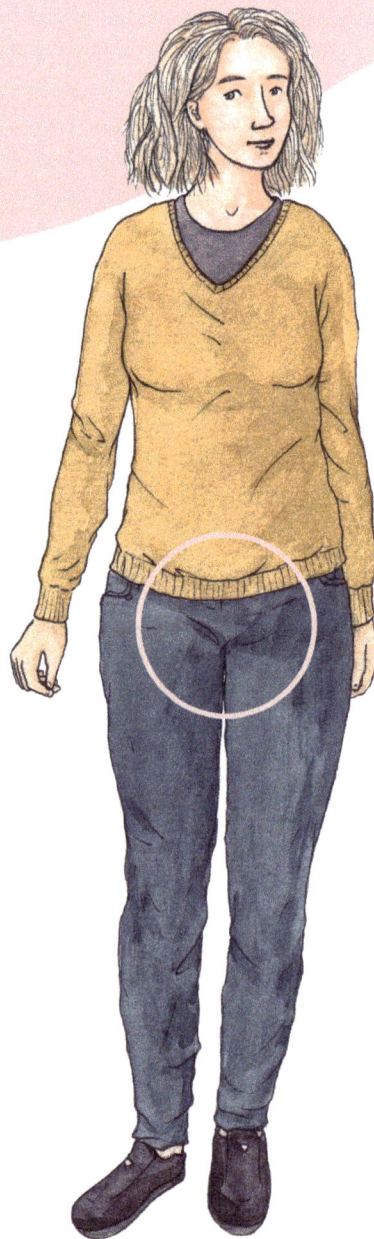

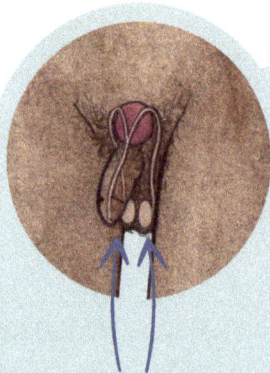

**THE SPERM ARE MADE HERE (IN THE TESTICLES).**

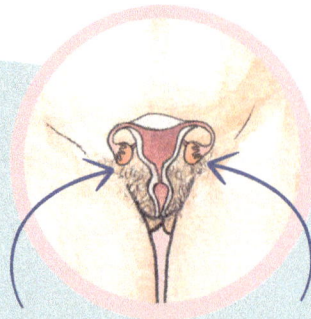

**THE EGGS LIVE HERE (IN THE OVARIES).**

The sperm will travel from the testicles through the penis and into the vagina. They use their wriggly tails to swim inside, where they might meet the egg.

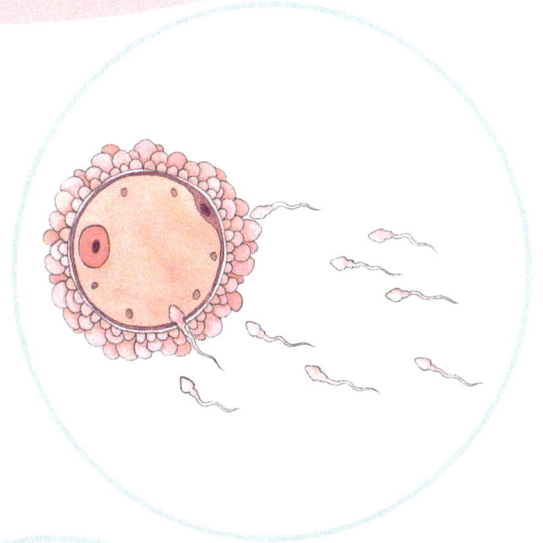

The sperm joins with the egg here.

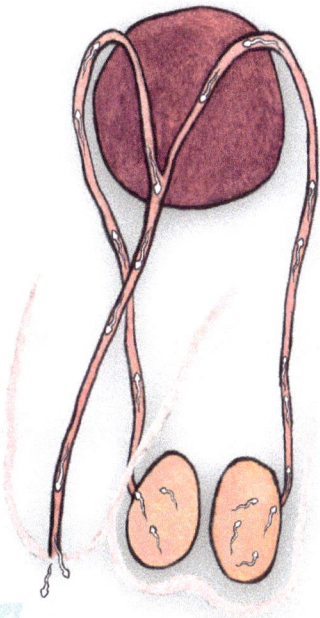

Sperm comes out here.

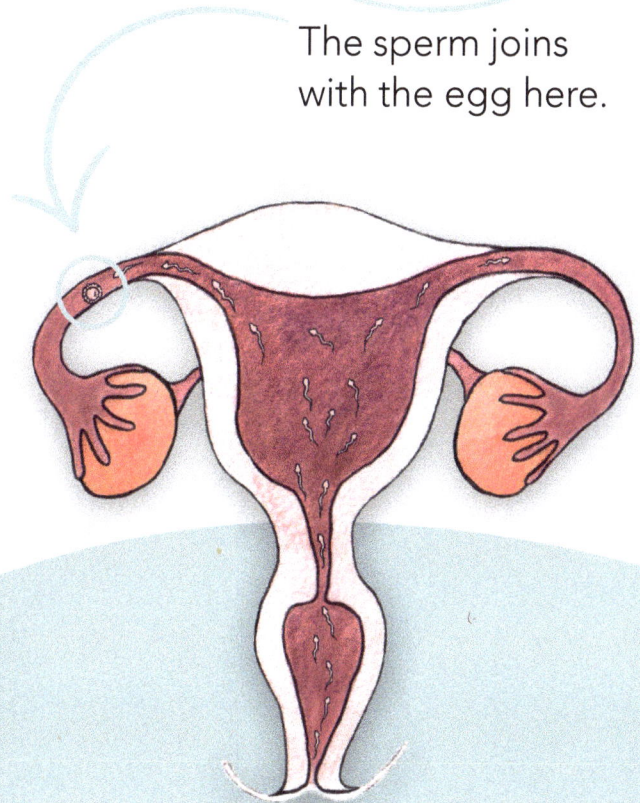

Sperm goes in here.

# 6 HOW DO THE SPERM AND EGG MEET?

## (SEX VERSION)

## THERE ARE LOTS OF WAYS TO MAKE A BABY.

A person with a vagina and a person with a penis can make a baby by having sex. The penis is placed inside the vagina. The sperm then travels from the testicles through the penis and into the vagina. The sperm swims into the uterus and fallopian tubes, where they might meet an egg. Sex is only for adults—not children!

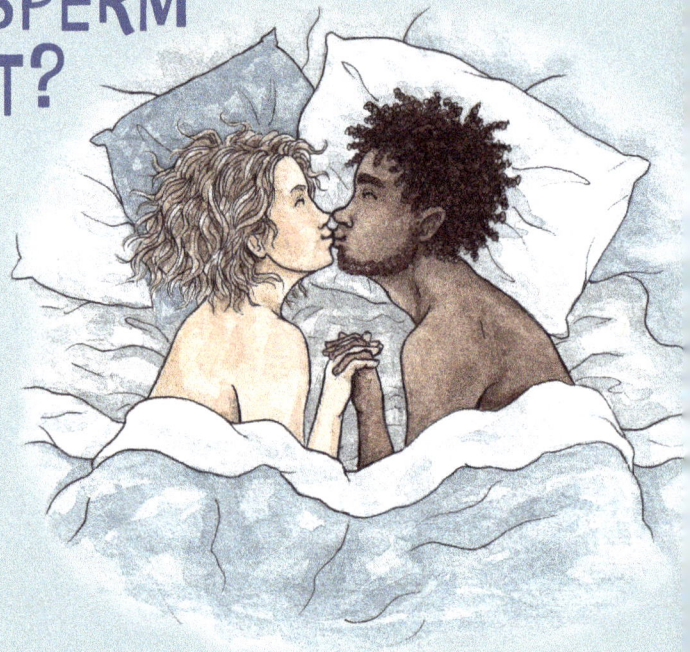

The sperm joins with the egg here, in the fallopian tubes.

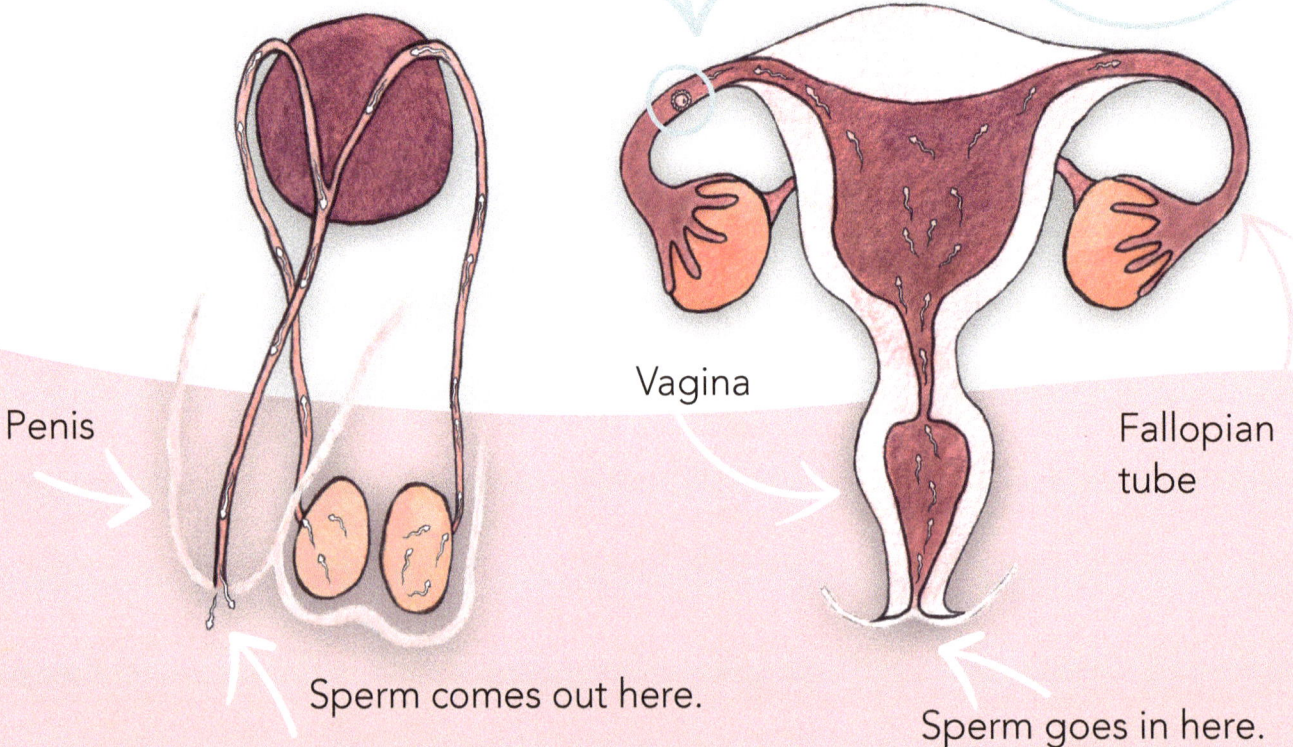

Penis

Sperm comes out here.

Vagina

Fallopian tube

Sperm goes in here.

# CAN BABIES BE MADE iN OTHER WAYS?

**7**

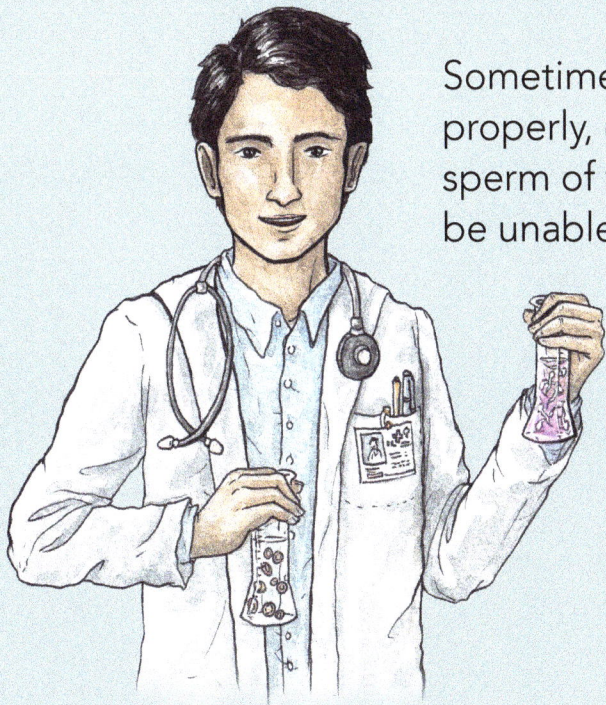

Sometimes, the sperm or egg might not work properly, or a person might not have an egg or sperm of their own. Alternatively, a person might be unable to grow a baby inside their body.

To get around these problems, someone might give them an egg or sperm, or offer to grow a baby inside their own uterus for them.

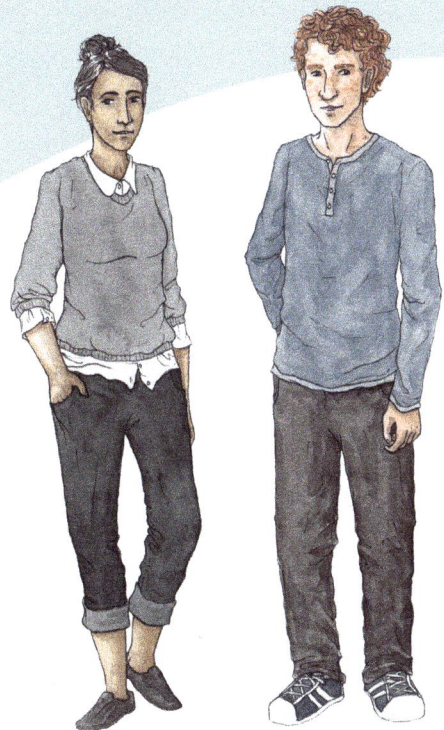

A doctor can help by placing the sperm inside the uterus. They may need to help the sperm and egg join together (this can happen inside or outside the body!).

Pictured are some of the special equipment doctors might use when helping people make a baby.

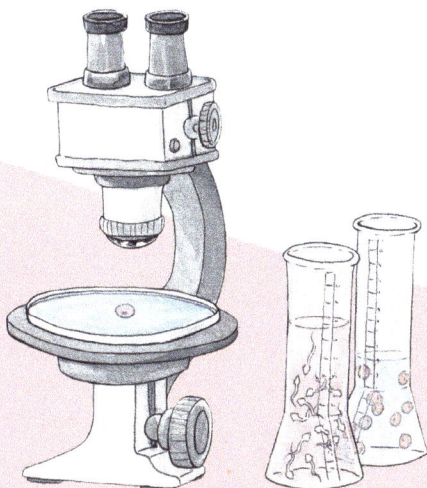

Some people might need special medicine to help them make a baby.

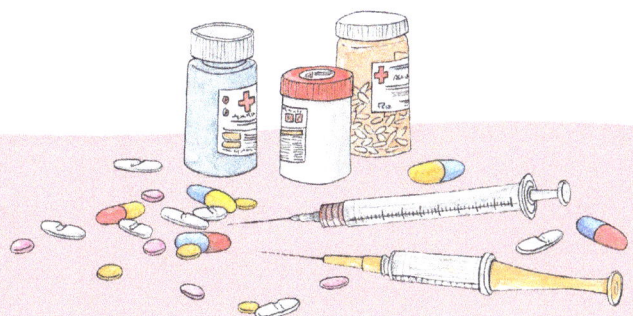

# 8  HOW DOES THE BABY COME OUT?

## THERE ARE TWO WAYS FOR A BABY TO COME OUT.

When it is time for the baby to come out, the person growing the baby inside them will start to feel pains in their stomach and back. Their uterus will get tight and then relax, get tight and then relax—this back-and-forth process helps them to push the baby out. This is called 'labour'.

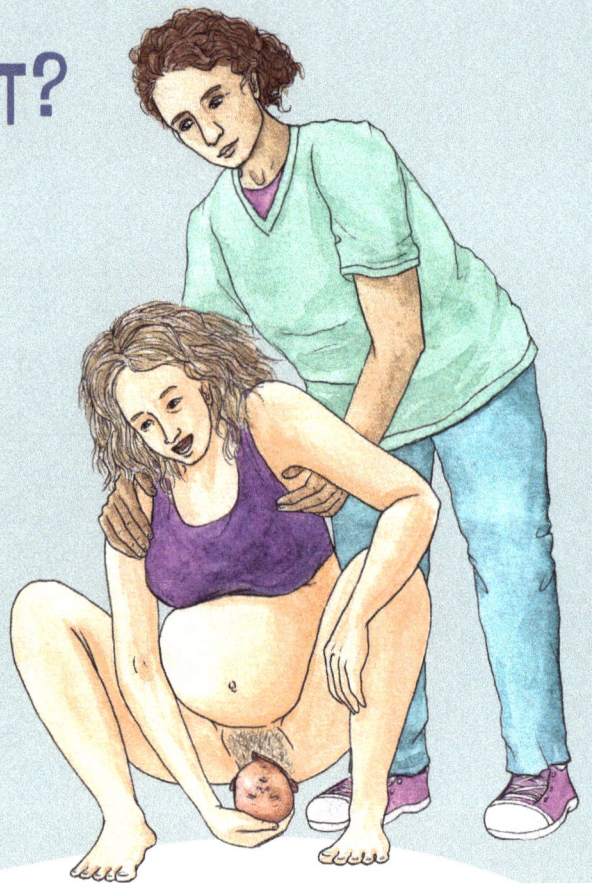

When the baby is ready to come out, the person will push it out of their vagina. The vagina will stretch to let the baby out. This is called a 'vaginal birth'.

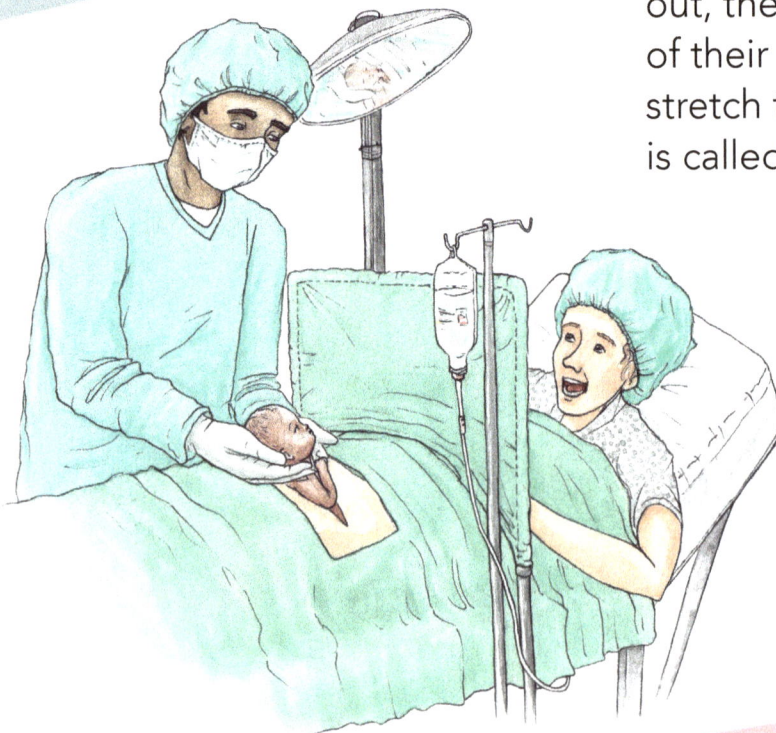

Some people need help to get the baby out. If this is the case, a doctor will cut a small hole in their tummy, take the baby out, and then close the hole. This is called a 'caesarean birth'.

# ABOUT THE AUTHOR

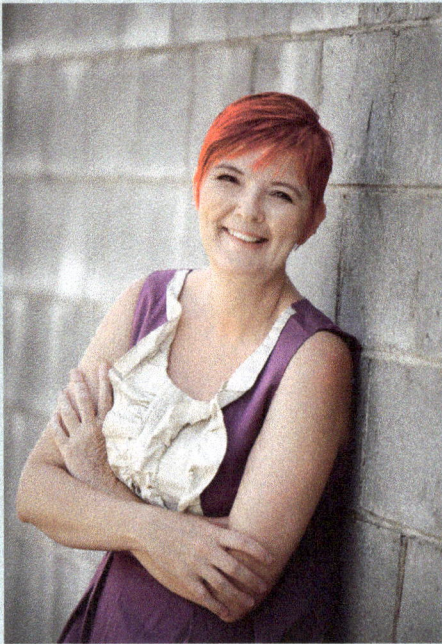

**Cath Hakanson** has been talking to clients about sex for the past 25 years as a nurse, midwife, sex therapist, researcher, author and educator. She's spent the past 15 years trying to unravel why parents (herself included) struggle with sex education. Her solution was to create Sex Ed Rescue, an online resource that simplifies sex education and helps parents to empower their children with the right information about sex, so kids can talk to them about anything, no matter what.

Cath has lived all over Australia but currently lives in Perth with her partner, 2 children, and ever-growing menagerie of pets. Despite having an unusual profession, she bakes, sews, and knits for sanity, collects sexual trivia, and tries really hard not to embarrass her children in public. Well, most of the time anyway!

*If you'd like to know more, please visit her online home at*

## SexEdRescue.com